GREEN TEA—THE ANCIENT SECRET FOR A HEALTHIER LIFE TODAY

Back in the 1970s, medical researchers noted that people who drank a perfectly natural but little-celebrated beverage seemed to have an extra measure of protection against cancer, heart attacks, strokes, infections, diarrhea, and other common ailments. It seemed almost too good to be true—but today, after decades of research, we know beyond a doubt that this "wonder substance" can:

- Protect against heart disease by regulating cholesterol and preventing platelets from forming deadly clots.
- Guard against the oxidants that destroy body tissue and damage the immune system.
- Prevent normal cells from turning cancerous.
- Suppress the formation and growth of tumors.
- Reduce the risk of developing cavities.

DISCOVER THE AMAZING BENEFITS OF THIS NATURAL HEALER

What else can green tea do? It fights deadly bacteria, including those that cause pneumonia, cholera, dysentery, and food poisoning, all without disturbing the "friendly" intestinal bacteria. It even combats the bacteria that cause bad breath! And it inhibits the action of viruses—including flu, herpes simplex, polio, and even part of the HIV virus—by preventing their attachment to cells. Green tea can also help you lose weight, because it actually suppresses the appetite and inhibits the accumulation of excess body fat!

GREEN TEA

FOR GOOD HEALTH AND LONG LIFE!

HEALTH CARE BOOKS FROM KENSINGTON

CANCER CURE   (1-57566-024-5, $12.00/$15.00)
The Complete Guide to Finding and Getting the Best Care There Is
by Gary L. Schine with Ellen Berlinsky, Ph.D.
Diagnosed with incurable cancer, Gary L. Schine was finally able to find the treatment that led him back to full recovery and perfect health. Now, in this inspiring and invaluable guide, he shows you how to take charge of your illness, your treatment, and your recovery.

HYPOGLYCEMIA   (1-57566-064-4, $13.00/$16.00)
The Disease Your Doctor Won't Treat
by Jeraldine Saunders and Dr. Harvey M. Ross
Do you suffer from unexplained tiredness, headaches, backaches, insomnia, depression, or memory loss? You may have hypoglycemia, a diet-related disease caused by sudden, rapid declines in levels of blood sugar. This landmark book contains a revolutionary new approach to treating hypoglycemia that will help you find the vital connection between what you eat and how you feel . . . physically and emotionally.

NO MORE RITALIN   (1-57566-126-8, $14.00/$18.00)
Treating ADHD Without Drugs
by Dr. Mary Ann Block
This breakthrough book shows why Ritalin may be extremely dangerous to your child's health and why the condition known as ADHD can and should be treated through safer and more effective means. Dr. Block's revolutionary method is based on the belief that you can't treat the problem until you identify the underlying causes of ADHD. Using actual case histories from her clinic, Dr. Block offers powerful evidence that a drug-free approach works.

GREEN
TEA

NADINE TAYLOR, M.S., R.D.

Kensington Books
Kensington Publishing Corp.
http://www.kensingtonbooks.com

KENSINGTON BOOKS are published by

Kensington Publishing Corp.
850 Third Avenue
New York, NY 10022

First Printing: January, 1998
10 9 8 7 6 5 4 3 2

Printed in the United States of America

To Barry,
my teacher, friend, true love,
and inspiration.

ACKNOWLEDGMENTS

Heartfelt thanks to John Szymanski for generously sharing his considerable knowledge of tea. Thanks to Dr. Yukihiko Hara, the world's foremost expert on green tea, for graciously taking the time to explain certain scientific concepts. Thanks also to Nina Ostrom Taylor for carefully reading the drafts and for always being the first to cheer when good things happen. And, of course, thanks to Barry Fox for being my guiding light.

Contents

CHAPTER 9

CHAPTER 10

Foreword

As a physician, I have seen many people suffer from serious diseases. Although there is much that modern medicine can do to help, it's clearly better to prevent illness in the first place, rather than try to treat it after the fact. Thanks to studies pouring in from hospitals and laboratories the world over, we know that one of the best preventive measures is a healthful diet—of which green tea can be an important part.

I've been impressed by the reports showing that green tea can help reduce one's risk of developing heart disease and certain forms of cancer, as well as help prevent or delay the onset of several other ailments. And with oxidation emerging as a leading cause of the physical and mental decline associated with aging, it's gratifying to learn that this inexpensive and tasty drink exhibits strong antioxidant properties.

In *Green Tea,* Nadine Taylor has brought together a tremendous number of scientific studies that explain why drinking tea can lead to a healthier life. And reading this fascinating book—filled as it is with interesting information about the history of tea, the differences between the types of tea, the Japanese and Chinese tea ceremonies, and many other "tea tidbits"—is as pleasurable as it is educational.

I'm convinced: Green tea is in many ways like a medicine. If only I could turn it into a pill and carry it in my little black bag!

ERIC MILLER, M.D.

CHAPTER 1

Tea: A Steaming Cup of Medicine

Anywhere a person cultivates tea, long life will follow.
—EISAI,
Maintaining Health by Drinking Tea, 1211

Back in the 1970s, medical researchers were startled to discover that people who drank moderate amounts of a certain natural substance seemed to have greater protection against cancer, heart attacks, strokes, infections, diarrhea, dental caries, and a host of other ailments. During the next twenty-five years, as research was conducted by scientists around the world, it was proven that this "wonder substance" could:

- Enhance immune system function by guarding against the oxidants and free radicals that weaken the body's natural defensive system.
- Prevent normal cells from turning cancerous.
- Suppress the formation and growth of tumors.
- Help regulate cholesterol levels.
- Lower the risk of stroke by making blood platelets less "sticky."
- Help control blood pressure.

- Lower the risk of epileptic seizures in laboratory animals.
- Help control blood sugar levels.
- Assist in weight loss by blocking the breakdown of starch.
- Ward off viruses, fungi, and food-borne bacteria.
- Fight bacteria in the mouth that cause cavities and bad breath.
- Slow the aging process.

And there's more. Scientists studying 3,380 women over the age of fifty living in Tokyo were astonished to find that those drinking this substance lived longer than those who did not![1] And many other studies conducted at leading medical centers and universities the world over confirmed that drinking moderate amounts of this amazing substance could actually help to lengthen life.

The good news is that this "wonder drug" is readily available and remarkably inexpensive. You can buy it in your local grocery or health food store. And it tastes delicious! What is this "wonder drug"? It's *green tea*. That's right. The simple, delicious beverage that's served to you in Japanese restaurants has amazing medicinal properties.

The fact that green tea promotes good health will come as no surprise to the Chinese and Japanese people, who have been drinking it for thousands of years. In fact, a whole book on the health benefits of green tea was written in the year 1211, in which the monk Eisai stated, "Tea is a miraculous medicine for the maintenance of health. Tea has an extraordinary power to prolong life."

Yes, green tea has been considered a "medicine" in China for over 4,000 years, and was written about by both Dharma, the founder of Zen Buddhism, and Shen-Nung, the father of the study of medicinal herbs. For these and many other ancients, tea was considered "the divine elixir of the gods."

1. Sadakata, 1992.

What Is Tea?

Tea comes from the *Camellia sinensis* plant, a cousin of the flowering camellia bushes that many people grow in their gardens. At one time, botanists thought there were two distinct varieties of tea: *Camellia sinensis*, which originated in China, thrived in the cool climate of the higher elevations, and produced small leaves about 3 inches long and 1 inch wide, and *Camellia assamica*, which was native to India and did well in semitropical climates, where it produced large leaves that could grow to be 10 inches long and 4 inches wide. But recently botanists concluded that, despite the obvious differences in these two plants, they actually belonged to the same species—*Camellia sinensis*.

The Real Thing

Although just about any drink made by combining hot water and leaves, flowers, or roots is commonly referred to as "tea," true tea is made only from the leaves and buds of the *Camellia sinensis* bush. Herbal tea, then, is not really tea at all.

Tea is an evergreen shrub that, when allowed to grow wild, produces fragrant white blossoms in the spring. These blossoms eventually form a fruit containing one to three small seeds. In order to reproduce, the tea plant must be cross-pollinated with another tea plant, and during this process genes and chromosomes are exchanged. Just as in animals, the baby tea plant winds up with some of the characteristics of one parent, and some of the other, as well as some from earlier ancestors that may have been dormant. Thus every tea plant is completely unique.

As in any group, there are always a few superachievers in a field of tea plants and one that looks no different from its neighbor might be able to produce twice as many high-quality tea leaves. Tea planters don't like to be at the mercy of random genetics, however, so they usually gather the seeds from their superior plants and cross-fertilize them with each other. Or they may "clone" a particular bush through a process called *layering*, in which the end of a branch that is still growing on the bush is buried. Once this branch establishes roots, it is cut away from the "mother" bush and continues to grow on its own. This way a bush can be exactly reproduced many times.

In the wild, a tea bush will become a 15–30-foot tree, surrounded by its offspring of little tea plants, but the cultivated tea plant is usually kept to a height of 3–5 feet for ease in plucking. Because its tender leaves can be easily scorched by the sun, tea is often planted among specially selected shade trees.

"King Tea Tree"

The largest tea tree in the world was discovered in 1939, growing wild in China's Yunnan province. At an estimated 1,700 years old, it was more than 100 feet high and the diameter of its trunk was greater than 1 yard.[2]

Plucking the Leaves

The part of the plant used for making tea is found in the uppermost section of the shoots, where the young, tender new leaves and buds are found. The development of these new buds and leaves is called the *flush*. For superior tea, harvesters pluck either the bud or the bud plus the youngest leaf, while for good to average tea, they take the bud and the top *two* leaves. "Coarse

2. Pratt, p. 212.

plucking," which results in average to below average tea, may consist of the bud, top two leaves, and the older leaf below them, plus some of the twig.

It's interesting to note that, even in our superindustrialized age, one plucking "tool" continues to outdo them all—human fingernails. Believe it or not, the majority of the world's tea plucking is still done by hand! Even in Japan or Taiwan, where some of the world's most complex electronics and machinery are manufactured, fine teas are *never* machine plucked. And with good reason—tea harvesting machinery tends to be indiscriminate and harsh, ripping off and crushing not just the bud and top one or two leaves, but also coarser leaves, twigs, and anything else that gets in its way. This rough handling encourages the onset of fermentation, something to be avoided at all costs in green tea production.

Tea—A Scent-ual Experience

"Freshly plucked tea leaf has the same spicy smell as the growing leaf, resembling that of ginger root or the concentrated smell of hay with the acrid part predominating. As withering proceeds, the leaf develops a marked fruity smell, as of apples. During the first ten minutes or so of rolling, the fruity smell is accentuated and includes the smell of pears. . . . Freshly fired tea has a smell of burnt toast and also a caramel smell of burnt sugar. . . ."

—C. R. Harler, *The Culture and Marketing of Tea*

Once the leaves have been plucked, they are whisked off for processing. The way the leaves are processed—whether they are withered, steamed, rolled, fermented, dried, or a combination of these methods—has everything to do with the kind of tea that's being manufactured.

Green, Black, or In Between?

There are three major kinds of tea—green, black and "other," such as oolong—each processed quite differently. To make black tea, the fresh tea leaf is withered by exposure to the air, and is broken and left to ferment after picking. Oolong tea is treated similarly, but the withering process is much shorter, resulting in a partially fermented leaf. For green tea, the leaf is not fermented at all. Instead, it is steamed immediately after harvesting to stop the fermentation process, then rolled and dried.

Who-Long?

Oolong tea, a marriage of the qualities of green and black teas, is sometimes referred to as "the champagne of teas" because of its distinctive taste. Its name comes from the Chinese *wu-lung,* which means "black dragon."[3]

More than 2.75 million metric tons of dried tea are manufactured every year, approximately 72% of it as black tea, 23% as green tea, and only 4%[4] as other tea.[5] Why does the world consume so much more black tea than green tea? One reason comes from the British tea importers themselves back in the seventeenth and eighteenth centuries. Green tea looked rather anemic to them, so the tea importers tried to give it more color by adding lead filings, chopped willow, elm leaves, and gypsum. Not surprisingly, those who drank this concoction became ill. Not realizing that it was the additives that made them sick, the British concluded that green tea was unhealthy because it wasn't "cooked" long enough!

3. Pratt, p. 225.
4. Graham, 1992.
5. Tea Council of the USA and International Tea Committee, London.

World Tea Production (1995)[6]

Total dry weight of tea measured in thousands of tons

Black Tea	1,993
Green Tea	624
Other Tea	135
TOTAL	**2,752**

Polyphenols, the Powerful Health Promoters

The manufacturing methods used in making black, oolong, and green tea not only alter the taste, aroma, and quality of the finished brew, but also change the way tea can affect your health. That's because unfermented green tea leaves contain much larger amounts of a group of potent health promoters called *polyphenols,* which are chemically changed during the fermentation of black and oolong teas.

Polyphenols are naturally occurring chemical compounds found in certain fruits and vegetables, potatoes, garlic, and a few other foods. A subgroup of the polyphenols—the *catechins* (pronounced "CAT-i-kins")— are particularly powerful disease fighters and potent antioxidants that have a host of beneficial effects, from preventing food spoilage to halting the progression of cancer. Catechins are found in wine, *Ginkgo biloba* leaves, and pine bark, but appear in the greatest quantity in fresh tea leaves.

The way the tea leaf is processed greatly affects the catechin content of the finished tea. For example, the catechin content of green tea is an impressive 15–30% of the tea's dry weight. Oolong, on the other hand,

6. Tea Council of the USA and International Tea Committee, London.

contains just 8–20% catechins, while black tea brings up the rear with only 3–10%.[7] What happens during the processing of oolong and black teas that "kills off" so many catechins? Well, it all begins in the tea field, as soon as the leaf is plucked from the plant.

Tea leaves contain an enzyme called *polyphenol oxidase*. When the leaf is plucked, this enzyme combines with oxygen (a process called *oxidation*) and begins to change the structure of the catechins. In the manufacturing of green tea, the number one goal is to prevent as much oxidation as possible. Some, of course, is inevitable. But the application of heat inactivates the enzyme, so the trick is to get the freshly plucked leaf from the field to a heat source as quickly as possible. That's why time is of the essence in green tea manufacturing: Once the leaf has been plucked, the race begins!

When manufacturing green tea, growers rush the leaves from the field to the factory, being careful not to bruise or break them, since that would speed up the oxidation process. At the factory, the leaves are steamed, pan-fired, or roasted to stop the enzyme-driven changes and preserve as many catechins as possible. Then they are rolled, twisted, and dried thoroughly. The beverage made from these tea leaves is clear light green to light golden brown in color, with a refreshing, slightly bitter, but smooth taste.

Black tea undergoes a completely different kind of processing. The leaves are plucked, but instead of being rushed to a heat source, they are spread on trays or racks and left to wither in the sun for 18–24 hours. During this time, one-third to one-half of their weight evaporates. Then the leaves are rolled and twisted in order to break down the cell walls and *accelerate* the oxidation of the catechins (exactly the opposite of what is done in green tea manufacturing).

7. Mitsui Norin Co., Ltd.

Green tea is produced in a four-step process:

- *Steaming or pan-firing* immediately after harvesting to kill the fermentation enzymes. This also makes the leaves soft and pliable.
- *Rolling*, either by hand or machine, on heated trays to reduce the moisture content.
- *Twisting*, which helps adjust the water content.
- *Drying*, during which the leaves are rolled, shaped, and styled.

Withering and twisting causes leaves to *ferment*, and during this process, the catechins are oxidized into more complex compounds called *thearubigens* and *theaflavins*. These compounds give black tea its characteristic color, aroma, and taste. In the final stage, the leaves are fired, which stops the fermentation and reduces the moisture content. Black tea produces a dark reddish-brown brew with a bittersweet taste and a rich, appealing aroma. The longer the leaves have been fermented, the darker the color and the less astringent the resulting tea.

Processing Black Tea

As with green tea, the making of black tea requires four major steps:

- *Withering*, in which leaves are spread on trays in the sun to soften and dry for 18–24 hours.
- *Rolling*, which breaks apart the cells in the leaf and releases enzymes which will act on the catechins.
- *Fermenting*, when enzymes and oxygen transform catechins into thearubigens and theaflavins.
- *Firing*, which stops the fermentation process and dries the leaves.

Keeping the Polyphenols in Green Tea

Protecting the polyphenols from oxidation is the most important part of the green tea manufacturing process. The leaves must be picked and rushed to the processing plant, where the oxidizing enzymes are stopped dead. The next step depends on where the leaves are being processed:

- In *China*, the tea leaves are rapidly pan-fired or roasted over wood or charcoal.
- In *Japan*, they are steamed for 20–50 seconds in large rotating cylinders.
- In *India*, they are rotated in heated cylinders for 7–10 minutes.

Then the tea is twisted and dried until the moisture content is reduced to about 3%. If done correctly, the processed green tea should be light yellow-green with absolutely no oxidation of the polyphenols.[8]

Whether the leaves are steamed, pan-fired, or rotated in heated cylinders doesn't seem to matter as far as taste or quality is concerned. The important thing is to stop the action of the oxidation of the polyphenols and any good heat source will do that. Roasting, however, gives a distinctly smoky, nut-like flavor that makes green tea taste like a completely different beverage.

To make oolong tea, manufacturing methods from both green and black tea are combined. The fresh leaves are spread out in large, flat baskets and left to wither in the sun for four to five hours. These baskets are shaken every so often to bruise the edges of the leaves, ensuring that more oxidation will occur at the edge of the leaves than in their centers. When the leaves are about half fermented, they are fired to stop the process and reduce moisture content. Then they are rolled, twisted, and dried.

8. Joy, 1986; Forster, 1990.

The Wondrous Catechins

For thousands of years, the Chinese have claimed that drinking tea is good for your health, both mentally and physically. But only recently have scientists been able to investigate these claims by isolating the components of tea and putting them to the test in laboratory experiments.

Curiosity about the effect of green tea on human health was first aroused in the 1970s. Epidemiologists noticed that people living in the Shizuoka Prefecture, an area in central Japan where green tea is grown and consumed in great quantities, had a much lower rate of death from stomach cancer than people living elsewhere in Japan.[9] This low death rate was very significant because stomach cancer was (and still is) the most prevalent form of cancer in Japan.

Once scientists began to study the people who lived in the Shizuoka Prefecture, they were surprised to discover that, not only did they die less often of stomach cancer, their death rates from *all types of cancers* were significantly lower. Curious and excited, the scientists conducted exhaustive studies of the population. The only major difference they could find was the people who lived in the Shizuoka Prefecture drank significantly more green tea than people living in areas with higher rates of cancer.[10]

Polyphenols? Flavonoids? Catechins?

As you read about green tea in books and magazines, you'll come across several related health terms. Although often used interchangeably, they have different meanings.

Polyphenols are naturally occurring compounds that act as powerful antioxidants.

---

9. Oguni, 1992.
10. Oguni, 1991.

There are many types of polyphenols, including the *flavonoids* found in green tea, fruits, and vegetables. (The flavonoids are also called bioflavonoids.)

Catechins are a particular kind of flavonoid found in tea, especially green tea. They're sometimes called green tea polyphenols.

Tea researchers usually talk about five types of catechins:

gallocatechin (GC)
epicatechin (EC)
epigallocatechin (EGC)
epicatechin gallate (ECg)
epigallocatechin gallate (EGCg), the most potent of the catechins

We will examine these more closely in Chapter 3.

Everybody drinks tea in Japan, and most of it is green. But they *really* drink it in the Shizuoka Prefecture, since acres and acres of tea grow right there, practically in the backyard. This easy accessibility makes for almost continual sipping throughout the day. The water is always boiling, and just-picked tea leaves are often added to the teapot to refresh the brew.

When studying black tea drinkers around the world, scientists didn't see the same dramatic cancer-protective effects as they saw in Shizuoka. But why not? they wondered. What did green tea have that black tea didn't have? The answer was clear—more catechins. Catechins make up as much as 30% of the dry weight of green tea leaves, but only 3–10% of black tea. So the scientists went back to their laboratories determined to prove (or disprove) the theory that the catechins in green tea were the miracle substance that could help prevent cancer.

In order to use the green tea leaf with maximum efficiency in tests on laboratory animals, researchers used a scientific process to extract its catechins and condense them into a powdered form. This powder could then be mixed with the food or drinking water or diluted and injected into the skin. Since the catechins were first isolated and tested, thousands of studies of their physiological effects have been conducted. And the results have been nothing short of astounding. As you will see in the chapters to come, *green tea protects against many of the most dangerous and deadly diseases plaguing humankind today*. And no matter how much green tea you may drink, there are literally *no adverse side effects*.

Other Health-Promoting Ingredients in Green Tea

In addition to the catechins, green tea contains these health promoters:

Flavonols—which (like the catechins) are a subgroup of the flavonoids known for their strong antioxidant properties. They help trap and destroy free radicals, singlet oxygen, and peroxides, keeping them from destroying body tissue. They also work together with vitamin C to help strengthen blood vessel walls.

Vitamin C—which helps to reduce stress, fight infection, and strengthen the immune system.

Vitamin B complex—which aids in the metabolism of carbohydrates.

Vitamin E—which has antioxidant properties and helps retard aging.

Fluoride—which helps to harden tooth enamel, thus preventing cavities.

But before we explore the "green tea miracle" any further, let's take a look at the origins of tea itself and how it spread throughout the world as a comforting and health-promoting beverage.

CHAPTER 2

The Story of Tea

There is a great deal of poetry and fine sentiment in a chest of tea.

—RALPH WALDO EMERSON,
Letters and Social Aims

Tea has been enjoyed for nearly 5,000 years, and from the very start it was found it to be a delicious, comforting beverage that was both medicinal and pleasing to the senses. The Chinese Emperor Shen-Nung, known as the "Divine Healer," is credited with discovering this delightful brew. Legend has it that some tea leaves blew into a pot of water that the Emperor was boiling, and lo and behold, a new beverage was born![1] Shen-Nung also produced the first written record of tea in his medical book, the *Pen Ts'ao*, written in 2737 B.C. In it, the Chinese ruler noted that tea "quenches thirst. It lessens the desire for sleep. It gladdens and cheers the heart."[2]

Another legend explaining tea's origins involves Dharma, the father of Zen Buddhism. According to legend, Dharma traveled from India to China in A.D. 520. There, he demonstrated the Zen art of meditation

1. Tea Council of the USA.
2. Schapira, p. 145.

to the Chinese by sitting in front of a wall for nine years. But one unfortunate day he dozed off, and when he awoke he was so angry with himself that he cut off his eyelids to make sure he would never sleep again. The bloody eyelids fell to the ground and became a tea plant, from which a beverage that lessened sleepiness could be made.[3]

The real origins of tea probably lie with the aboriginal natives who lived in what is now Southeast Asia. Tea grows wild there, as it does from the southernmost province of China to the border of Vietnam. The early natives undoubtedly made a medicine from the tea leaves by boiling them in water and drinking the resulting infusion.

Before it was ever used as a beverage, though, tea was considered a food in several parts of the world. In Burma, for example, tea leaves were pickled and eaten as a salad. In Siam, steamed tea leaves were eaten with dried fish, pig fat, garlic, salt, and oil. In Kashmir, a popular dish consisted of tea leaves mixed with salt, anise, and red potash. And in Tibet, tea was combined with barley meal, goat's milk butter, and salt, all of which were mixed to the consistency of a thick paste and eaten for breakfast.[4]

The first credible record of the cultivation of tea was written in A.D. 350 by Kuo P'o, who defined it as: "a beverage . . . made from the leaves by boiling."[5] At this time tea was highly regarded as a medicine, although not yet as an everyday beverage. Written records of the time note that tea was used to cure a wide range of digestive disorders and nervous conditions, and was also made into a paste to be applied externally to cure the pains of rheumatism.[6] But the desire for tea was growing rapidly, and soon just plucking from the nearby trees

3. Schapira, p. 146.
4. Schapira, p. 148.
5. Pratt, p. 199
6. Schapira, p. 149

was not enough. So began the deliberate cultivation of tea plants in the hills of Szechwan.

By the fifth century A.D., the practice of drinking tea for pleasure (in addition to its medicinal uses) was common in many areas of China. Most farmers of the era used at least part of their land to cultivate tea, and just about every peasant grew a few bushes for private use. But the cultivation, manufacturing, and preparation of tea was still quite primitive, with methods passed along from generation to generation almost entirely by word of mouth or by example.[7]

Tea leaves were first carried west by Turkish traders who bartered with the Chinese at the Mongolian border. The Turks traded tea with others along their many and varied routes, and soon tea's reputation as a delicious beverage spread to nearby lands. By 780, tea trading had become so popular that the Chinese government levied a tax on it.

In that same year, the first authentic written account of the preparation and manufacture of tea was presented in the book called *Ch'a Ching (Classic of Tea)*, written by Lu Yu,[8] a poet and scholar who became the patron saint of tea. In his three-volume work, Lu Yu described everything that was then known about tea: the origins of the tea plant, the varieties of tea, the methods of tea cultivation and production, the benefits of tea drinking, and precise instructions for brewing and serving tea. He even devised a ceremonial way to drink tea, and his version of "afternoon tea" required no less than twenty-four objects, which were used to measure, prepare, and finally serve this distinguished beverage! From that time on, *Ch'a Ching* became the tea "bible," and Lu Yu became the ultimate authority on the subject of tea.

During the Sung Dynasty (960–1280), the rise of tea continued. At this time, flavoring it with pickle juice,

7. Schapira, p. 150.
8. Weatherstone, p. 2.

onions, ginger, and orange was all the rage. Whipped tea was also fashionable, with powdered tea leaves beaten to a froth in hot water with a small bamboo whisk.[9] Whipped powdered tea (matcha) is the form still used today in the Japanese tea ceremony.

As tea's popularity continued to soar, the Chinese government decided to open up regular tea trading across the Mongolian border. For the first time ever, tea was exported to Tibet, although the process of getting it there wasn't easy! Porters, who were treated as human "beasts of burden," had to carry 300-pound loads on their backs while hiking through steep mountain passes, some of which were 5,000 feet high. The weight of these packs was so unbearable that the porters had to put opium behind their ears to kill the pain and keep themselves from collapsing.[10]

Tea arrived in Japan in 729, courtesy of Buddhist monks who had been studying in China. At a Buddhist scripture reading that lasted for four days, the Chinese Emperor Shomu gave powdered tea to the 100 monks in attendance.[11] The monks found the tea useful not only as a medicine but as a "pick-me-up" that helped to keep them from dozing during long meditation sessions. Upon returning to Japan, the monks enthusiastically began to plant tea shrubs and to practice their own version of Lu Yu's tea ceremony as a spiritual exercise. Over time, the beverage that "relieved fatigue, strengthened the will and lifted the spirit,"[12] began to find its way into high society. Tea's high status was finally secured in 794, when the Emperor Kammu insisted that the new Imperial Palace, currently under construction, have its own tea garden.[13]

The monk Eisai (who was famous for introducing Zen to Japan) promoted tea drinking in his book *Main-*

9. Schapira, p. 152.
10. Weatherstone, pp. 2–3.
11. Schapira, p. 154.
12. Yokoyama, p. 2.
13. Schapira, p. 154.

taining Health by Drinking Tea, written in 1211. In it, he described a tea ceremony based on Buddhist principles and spread the word about the spiritual and health-promoting properties of tea. But by the beginning of the fourteenth century, tea had become more popular as a pleasure than as a conduit to physical or spiritual fulfillment. It was enthusiastically adopted by the Japanese nobility as a luxury, and a favorite activity was participation in "tea tournaments." While relaxing on leopard or tiger skins in spacious tea pavilions, the guests would taste different teas and guess where they came from. Whoever guessed right was given one of the many treasures that decorated the pavilion. Depending on the amounts of tea offered, these tournaments were referred to as "10 bowl," "50 bowl," or even "100 bowl" events.[14]

Tea's popularity endured, and in the sixteenth century one of its greatest fans was Japan's mightiest warlord, Toyotomi Hideyoshi. He was so enamored of tea that he practiced the tea ceremony regularly and gave what may have been the largest tea party in history for all of his soldiers on the night before an important battle. He even insisted that his Tea Master, a man by the name of Senno Rikyu, accompany him to the battlefield and set up a portable tea house before each battle. There both sides could meet for discussion and meditation. Senno Rikyu (now known as the greatest of all Japanese tea masters) eventually devised seven rules for the tea ceremony which incorporated a philosophic bent that has not been matched to this day. The ceremony emphasized harmony, simplicity, love of nature, purity, politeness, the proper attitude, and a reverence for the aesthetic.[15] Thanks to its simplicity and the fact that no fancy equipment was needed, the tea ceremony became accessible to the middle class and not just the

14. Pratt, p. 25.
15. Schapira, p. 156.

rich. This ensured that the use of tea in Japan would become almost universal.

Western countries, already interested in silks, spices, dyes, and other products from the Far East, were intrigued in 1559 by the first mention of tea in a European book called *Voyages and Travels*. But the trip to China via land routes was long, difficult, and dangerous, so little tea was imported. Spain and Portugal were the first to reach the Orient by sea, sailing around the tip of Africa to bring tea, as well as other exotic goods, back to Lisbon and the Spanish peninsula.

What's in a Name?

Throughout the world, tea is referred to by any of four different names[16]:

Cha—This is the Cantonese word for tea, the name that was used on the overland trade routes from the time of the earliest exportation. It is now also a part of the Persian and Hindi languages.

Chai—A corruption of the word *cha*, chai is still the word for tea in Russia and in some areas of India, Afghanistan, and Iran.

Tay—The Dutch learned this name for tea (spelled *t'e*) when trading with the Fukien province across the strait from Taiwan, where the Amoy dialect is spoken. They introduced "tay" to Europe, where it was pronounced as such in England until 1712. The Irish still call it "tay."

Tea—British corruption of *t'e*.

In 1595, a Dutch navigator named Jan Hugo van Lin-Schooten published an account of his travels to Japan, including descriptions of the Japanese tea ceremony and the beautiful tea artifacts they used. As a direct result of Lin-Schooten's book, the Dutch set up a trading

16. Republic of Tea, p. 61.

station for Oriental goods on Java, and by 1602 more than sixty ships had made the voyage to and fro. So it was that in 1610 the first shipments of tea arrived in Europe via Dutch sailing ships.[17]

A Subtle Reminder

Father Alvaro Samedo, a Portuguese Jesuit who spent twenty-two years at the Chinese court in the 1500s, reported that offering tea to a guest was a sign of honor, but serving him a third cup was a hint to leave![18]

Before the seventeenth century, tea could be found in Europe only at court or in the homes of aristocrats. But that all changed in 1657 when, for the first time, tea was served to the English public at Garraway's Coffee House in London. Thomas Garraway, the proprietor, posted a sign listing the virtues of his establishment's exciting new beverage, which was soon to become the national drink of the British Isles:

> It maketh the body active and lusty.
> It helpeth the Headache, giddiness and
>   heavyness thereof.
> It removeth the obstructions of the Spleen.
> It is very good against the Stone and Gravel,
>   cleaning the kidneys and Uriters, being
>   drank with Virgins Honey instead of
>   Sugar.
> It taketh away the difficulty of breathing,
>   opening obstructions . . .
> It vanquisheth heavy dreams, easeth the
>   Brain and strengtheneth the
>   Memory.''[19]

17. Schapira, p. 161.
18. Ibid.
19. Ukers, 1935.

Russia got into the act at the end of the seventeenth century by opening trade with China for tea. Caravans of 200–300 camels carrying four chests of tea apiece crossed the great Gobi desert, trudged through Mongolia, then proceeded all the way across the endless Russian plains before reaching their destination. At a camel's leisurely pace, a round trip took about three years![20]

The World's Biggest Teapot

Russians took wholeheartedly to drinking tea during the eighteenth century. To keep hot water constantly at hand, they invented the samovar—a gigantic teapot and water heater with a 40-cup capacity. Tea was made by mixing one part tea leaves with three parts hot water, and adding lemon or jam to taste. The Russians were fond of drinking their tea while holding a cube of sugar between the teeth. By continually sipping, they were able to keep their spirits up and their hunger pangs down as they waited for their one big meal of the day.[21]

Until 1689, all of England's tea was supplied by the Dutch. But as the demand became more widespread, England decided to get into the tea-importing business herself. The East India Company (which had been formed in 1600 in response to a steep rise in the Dutch price of pepper) began to import tea directly from China. Their ships, heavily armed to guard against pirates, set sail on the long and difficult voyage from London to China. In spite of the fact that it took an entire year to make the round trip, and despite the many ships lost at sea, the East India Company was able to monopolize England's tea trade with China for almost 150 years.

20. Weatherstone, p. 3.
21. Schapira, p. 165.

Deliverance

"Tea had come as a deliverer to a land that called for deliverance; a land of beef and ale, of heavy eating and abundant drunkenness; of gray skies and harsh winds; of strong-nerved, stout-purposed, slow-thinking men and women. Above all, a land of sheltered homes and warm firesides—firesides that were waiting—waiting, for the bubbling kettle and the fragrant breath of tea."

—Agnes Repplier, *To Think of Tea!*

During the seventeenth century, tea was introduced to just about every country in the West. Although at first it was eagerly embraced by all, the novelty wore off rather quickly for some nations. Germany, for example, had its fling with tea and then returned to its old favorite, beer. France quickly bypassed tea in favor of wine and coffee, as did Portugal and Spain. But Russia was never fickle. To this day, she continues her love affair with tea, probably because she shares a common border with China and has many tea plantations herself. And in Great Britain, of course, tea has become absolutely indispensable and is a vital part of the national culture.

Hooked on Tea

Dr. Samuel Johnson (1709–84), the famous British lexicographer, was quoted in *The Literary Magazine* describing himself as: "A hardened and shameless tea drinker who has, for twenty years, diluted his meals with only the infusion of this fascinating plant; whose kettle has scarcely time to cool; who with tea amuses the evening, with tea solaces the midnight, and with tea welcomes the morning."

Tea was also highly popular in the American colonies during the seventeenth and eighteenth centuries; that is, until Britain levied a stringent tea tax. The incensed Colonists expressed their disapproval by tossing chests of tea over the sides of English ships and into Boston Harbor during what became known as the Boston Tea Party. From that point on, two trends were firmly set in motion; the move toward American independence and the move toward adopting coffee as the national drink.

Time for a Spot of Tea

The custom of afternoon tea was created by Anna, Duchess of Bedford, around 1840. The aristocracy of the day were accustomed to eating a large breakfast, very little lunch, and a late supper. But Anna got hungry around 4:00 P.M. every day. To ward off "that sinking feeling," she started snacking on tea and sandwiches.[22] This pleasant diversion is still very much alive in the British Isles today.

Although coffee became the beverage of choice in the United States, many people still had an affinity for tea. Rather than deal with the British, however, the United States decided to enter the business of importing tea herself. Through the early 1800s, tea was still brought back from China on huge, full-bodied frigates that took forever to make the trip. But in 1841, the United States, demonstrating the ingenuity that was so typical of this young, fledgling country, came up with its own contribution to the tea importation business— the *clipper ship*.

With its narrow, knifelike form and concave bow, the clipper ships could slice cleanly through the water and make the trip to and from China in nearly half the time! These ships caught on quickly, not only with tea compa-

22. Pratt, p. 48.

nies in their native America, but with companies in Europe as well. Soon, even faster ships that could hold more than a million pounds of tea were put to use. The clipper ships could make it from China to London in just four months. This was especially important because in England (still the largest market for tea), the spring flush brought in the most money and reportedly made the finest and most delicious tea. To give the ship captains extra incentive, tea companies bestowed handsome rewards on the first to deliver this batch. A great competition sprang up among the captains of the clipper ships as they vied to be the first to bring in the new tea. Plucked at the end of April, the spring flush was usually processed, packed into the ships, and ready to sail by the end of May. Then the race was on! The first mighty clipper ship to make it back to London was well rewarded and received a hero's welcome from cheering throngs and hordes of newspaper reporters.

But the glamorous and glorious era of the clipper ships was to end abruptly in 1869 with the opening of the Suez Canal. Suddenly it was possible for steamer ships to make the trip to China in as little as forty-four days, making even the fastest clipper ships completely obsolete.

During the 1850s, China's stranglehold on the tea trade began to fade. A similar kind of tea plant was discovered growing wild in India, and England began to develop her own tea plantations there. In 1887, for the first time Britain imported more tea from India and Ceylon than from China, a sign of the times. Just thirteen years later, in 1900, China's exportation of tea had dropped dramatically. She would never be able to regain her prominence in the tea exportation business.

"On the Rocks" or "Straight Up"?

Iced tea was invented in 1904 by an Englishman named Richard Blechynden who had a tea stand at the

St. Louis World's Fair. He was promoting hot Indian tea, but an intense heat wave made the public pass right by his tea. Finally, in desperation, Blechynden poured the tea over glasses of ice just to get people to try it. Iced tea caught on instantly and a new beverage craze was born.[23]

Today, 80% of the tea that Americans consume is iced tea—which amounts to over 40 billion servings per year, or enough to fill 130,000 backyard swimming pools.[24]

The Discovery of Tea in India

In 1823, the English Major Robert Bruce, who was stationed in the Indian province of Assam, was given a hot cup of brew by some local natives. It was a drink they had made from the dried leaves of some nearby plants. Thinking that the drink tasted quite a bit like tea, Major Bruce asked to see the plants, and was surprised to discover tea trees growing wild. Bruce sent samples of the trees to the Botanical Gardens in Calcutta, where they were classified as plants from the same family as Chinese teas (*Camellia*), but a different species (*assamica*, rather than *sinensis*). Amazingly, the discovery was then ignored for the next nine years.

In 1832, Lieutenant Charlton of the Assam Light Infantry made a similar discovery, finding wild tea plants growing near his barracks. He also sent samples to the Botanical Gardens in Calcutta, but this time the East India Company got wind of the discovery. The tea company had been trying to find a way to grow tea somewhere within the British Empire so they wouldn't have to import it from any other country. Understandably, they preferred to be their own supplier of tea, possibly even selling it to others. India was the obvious choice

23. Pratt, p. 93.
24. The Tea Council of the USA.

for tea cultivation, since it was part of the British Empire and was home to acres of undeveloped land.

The East India Company had everything they needed to grow and sell tea—except the tea plants themselves. Lieutenant Charlton's find proved that tea, or tealike plants, could grow in India. Of course, they wanted "real" tea, which to them meant tea from China. So early in 1834, the East India Company sent their secretary, G. J. Gordon, to China to steal the seeds of tea plants. He also had orders to bring back some experienced tea makers that could teach the naïve British tea growers how to cultivate the plants and process the leaves for the manufacture of tea.

After several harrowing escapes, Gordon sent about 80,000 seeds back to India, from which 42,000 plants were germinated. Most of the plants died but a few took root, especially in the Assam area.

Seed from both the Chinese plants and the indigenous Indian tea plants were eventually sent to other areas of India, to Ceylon, Java, Sumatra, and even to Russia, where tea cultivation was established in Georgia.

How Did China Lose Her Place?

There are several reasons why China lost her centuries-old monopoly on the tea trade. Government, politics, drugs, and foreigners all played a part. But a lack of plain old business sense also contributed to China's downfall.

For a long time she had the perfect situation—tea thrived in the Chinese climate and soil, manufacturing was complex (and the Chinese weren't about to reveal their secrets!), and demand was greater than supply. So what went wrong? Basically, China failed to do three things:

- *Organize.* The Chinese methods of cultivation hadn't changed for centuries. Tea was still grown on small plots of land by individual farmers. Once the plantation-style cultivation of tea began in India, it could be produced much more cheaply. But China couldn't produce enough tea to compete with these new, lower prices.

- *Industrialize.* The British brought machines to their Indian plantations to perform many of the tea-processing chores. This saved a great deal of labor, money, and (especially) time. Just one machine could roll as many leaves as sixty men could in the same amount of time, and one large dryer could perform the work of thirty-five men.[25] The Chinese, however, continued to do everything by hand.

- *Advertise.* Because their tea had been sought-after for centuries, the Chinese must have believed it would always be so. They did nothing to promote their product or provide any reason for importers to make the lengthy and expensive trip halfway around the world. Then, when someone else came up with a tea that was not only closer in proximity but cheaper, they lost their customers in droves.

Who Produces Tea Today?

Only about thirty countries produce tea today, the principal sources being India, China, Kenya, and Sri Lanka. (*See* Table 1.) Tea is grown as far north as Georgia in southern Russia, and as far south as Argentina in South America.

Fewer than ten countries produce green tea, with the bulk of it originating in China. (*See* Table 2.) Japan runs a distant second, but only about 2% of its tea is actually exported, with 98% of the crop consumed by the Japanese themselves. Of its tiny export crop, the United States takes more than 80%.[26]

25. Weatherstone, p. 15.
26. Schapira, p. 214.

TABLE 1

Yields of Major Tea-Producing Countries (1995)

Total dry weight of tea, in thousands of tons

India	831
China	649
Sri Lanka	272
Kenya	270
Indonesia	147
Turkey	115
Japan	93
Bangladesh	52
South America	49
U.S.S.R.	17
Others	257
TOTAL	**2,752**

Source: Tea Council of the USA and International Tea Committee, London.

The World's Biggest Tea Drinkers

Tea is the world's most widely consumed beverage after water, although consumption varies greatly from country to country and from person to person. One individual may drink no tea at all, while another may drink as many as 20 cups a day. On a per capita basis, however, Ireland is home to those who drink the most tea, with the average person consuming more than 3 kilograms (close to 7 pounds) of dry tea per year. The British follow closely, with 2.53 kilograms. Surprisingly, Japan ranks only thirteenth on the tea consumer list (*see* Table 3), even though we think of the Japanese as being avid tea drinkers. (Figures are not available for China.)

TABLE 2

Green Tea–Producing Countries (1995)

Total dry weight of tea measured in thousands of tons

China	456
Japan	93
Indonesia	33
Vietnam	28
India	9
U.S.S.R.	3
Sri Lanka	1
Bangladesh	1
Total	**624**

Source: Tea Council of the USA and International Tea Committee, London.

> "Thank God for tea! What would the world do without tea? How did it exist? I am glad I was not born before tea."
> —The Reverend Sidney Smith, 1771–1845

TABLE 3

Tea Consumption in Selected Countries

In kilograms per capita, average for years 1993–95

Ireland	3.16
United Kingdom	2.53
Kuwait	2.52
Turkey	2.02
Syria	1.55
Hong Kong	1.48
Iran	1.32
Sri Lanka	1.29
Morocco	1.24
New Zealand	1.23
Tunisia	1.17
Egypt	1.04
Japan	1.03
Chile	0.97
Poland	0.87
Canada	0.47
USA	0.34

(Figures not available for China.)

Source: Tea Council of the USA and International Tea Committee, London.

Now that we know the story of that precious commodity called tea, let's take an in-depth look at how this delicious beverage can help us hold on to another precious commodity—good health.

CHAPTER 3

Combating Cancer

Green tea can't prevent every cancer, but it's the cheapest and most practical method for cancer prevention available to the general public.
— HIROTA FUJIKI, Chemist,
    National Cancer Center Research Institute,
    Tokyo, Japan

Everybody's worried about getting cancer—with good reason. One out of four of us will contact cancer, and one out of five of us will die from it. It's the biggest killer disease in America after heart disease, with doctors diagnosing more than one million new cases of cancer each year.[1] This stealthy killer can strike anyone—senior citizens, people in the prime of life, and even children. It can take hold in virtually any organ, and you may not even know you have it until it's too late. In many cases, the "cure" can seem worse than the disease. Most of us have known someone with cancer who has suffered through the horrors of radiation, chemotherapy, surgery, and other cancer treatments. It's best, of course, to find a way to keep cancer from settling in to begin with.

Despite its fearsome reputation, many (or even most) forms of cancer *can* be avoided. For example, an

1. American Cancer Society.

amazing 60% of cancers in women are believed to be *directly related to diet*, and could be prevented simply by changing one's eating habits. In men, a hefty 30–40% of all cancers might be avoided by changes in the diet. The National Cancer Institute has issued special dietary guidelines to help us avoid cancer, and it even backs a special "Designer Nutrient Program" that investigates the powers of cancer-fighting foods and nutrients such as garlic, gingko biloba, and echinacea. One of the more recent additions to their program is green tea.

How Does Cancer Start and Spread?

No one knows exactly what *causes* cancer, but most scientists believe that the disease develops in two stages, *initiation* and *activation*. During the *initiation stage*, healthy cells are exposed to substances called *initiators*. (Cigarette smoke, radiation, environmental pollutants, chemicals, pesticides, ultraviolet light, and dietary fat can all be initiators.) These initiators break into the cell and "hijack" its DNA, altering the "instruction manuals" that tell the cell how to behave. It's as if an evil new captain has stormed aboard ship, thrown the old captain overboard, and ordered the crew to rebuild the boat, turning a peaceful pleasure craft into a deadly, heavily armed raider.

Initiated cells may lie quietly in the body for weeks, months, or even years, causing no damage. But at some point they can become *activated*. Then they begin to multiply uncontrollably, forming a mass of new tissue called a *tumor*, which invades the surrounding healthy tissues and structures, using up nutrients and crowding out the healthy cells. Eventually the tumor, which serves no useful purpose, can destroy large amounts of healthy cells and tissue, causing devastation, disease, and possibly even death.

Dietary fat, obesity, asbestos, alcohol, smoked or cured meats, and charbroiled meats, among other things, can serve as cancer activators. Fat, one of the few foods that can initiate *and* promote cancer, has been directly linked to the development of breast, colon/rectal, and prostate cancers.[2]

Cancer's Seven Warning Signals

If you have any of these warning signs, or any other reason to suspect cancer, see your doctor:

- Change in bowel or bladder habits
- Unusual bleeding or discharge
- Thickening or lump in the breast or elsewhere
- Obvious change in wart or mole
- Nagging cough or hoarseness
- A sore that does not heal
- Indigestion or difficulty in swallowing

If you're in good health, your immune system will usually zero in on the initiated cells before they are activated and simply "blast them out of the water." But if your immune system has been weakened, or if it's overwhelmed by having to fight too many mutated cells at once, some cancer cells may slip by. Once they take "root" and form a tumor, the cancer process is well underway.

Luckily, many natural, readily available substances help fight both initiation and activation. Some of the most powerful of these protectors are the *antioxidants,* effective cancer inhibitors found in a wide variety of foods and supplements. Well-known antioxidants include *vitamin A* (and its plant form, *beta carotene*), *vitamin C, vitamin E,* the mineral *selenium,* the *bioflavonoids,* and the *polyphenols.*

You may be wondering why anything that is *anti*-oxygen is good for you—after all, the body must have

2. American Institute for Cancer Research.

a continuous supply of oxygen in order to survive. The antioxidants are not against oxygen per se; instead they work against *oxidation*. You're familiar with oxidation—it's the process that turns bananas black, makes bread stale, and causes metal to rust. This same process occurs in the body and is believed to be one of the biggest causes of disease.

Oxygen normally travels around the body in pairs. These pairs of oxygen molecules, which peacefully share electrons, are described as "O_2" by chemists. But sometimes, as a part of the body's metabolic reactions, a double molecule splits and becomes two separate oxygen molecules known as *singlet oxygen*.

Singlet oxygen is one of a group of substances called *free radicals*, highly reactive and unstable molecules. In the case of singlet oxygen, since it's been separated from its "other half," it's missing an electron. Like a lovesick teenager, singlet oxygen desperately wants to be paired up, so it races crazily through the body in search of an electron to replace the one it lost. Desperate to find an electron, it will greedily snatch one from another molecule, just like a needy girl stealing somebody else's boyfriend. Of course, the molecule that was robbed of an electron is now upset and it, in turn, steals some other molecule's electron. You can imagine how cells, tissues, organs, and entire body systems can be degraded and even destroyed if enough of this "electron snatching" goes on. That's why many scientists believe that free radicals are a major cause of both aging and disease.

Green Tea Antioxidants to the Rescue!

Fortunately, we have *antioxidants* to protect us against the dangerous free radicals, especially singlet oxygen. Found in abundance in fruits, vegetables, and grains, these natural substances are powerful weapons against cancer, heart disease, stroke, aging, and many other deadly conditions. The antioxidants neutralize the rampaging singlet oxygen and other free radicals, stabilizing or "quenching" them so that they no longer have the urge to "steal." The antioxidants not only protect the body from the damaging effect of free radicals, they can also protect each other from being oxidized and "used up."

Polyphenols are powerful antioxidants found in green tea, garlic, fruits, potatoes, and some varieties of nuts. They are especially effective because they work against cancer during both the intiation and activation stages. During the initiation stage they help neutralize carcinogens to prevent them from "hijacking" healthy cells. And during the activation state, the polyphenols can actually stop some forms of cancer in their tracks by preventing cancer cells from turning into tumors.

There are many kinds of polyphenols, with names like *caffeic acid, chlorogenic acid,* and *ellagic acid.* But the *catechins*—the polyphenols unique to green tea—may be the strongest and most remarkable of all.

The catechins were discovered when curious epidemiologists in the 1970s wondered why people living in Japan's Shizuoka Prefecture had much lower rates of cancer than other Japanese (including stomach cancer, the country's leading cause of death[3]). Their interest was further aroused by a comparison of the lung cancer rates in Japan to those of the United States. It seems that the Japanese smoked nearly *twice* as many cigarettes as Americans, but had only about *half* the amount of lung cancer. Not only that, the average Japanese person outlived the average American by 7.2 years!

Delving into the question of whether or not green tea protected against lung cancer, scientists at the Naylor Dana Institute for Disease Prevention in New York gave a green tea solution to a group of mice for two weeks. Then they injected the mice with NNK, a potent carcinogen found in cigarette smoke, three times a week

3. Oguni, 1989.

for the next ten weeks, while continuing with the green tea. A control group received the same injections, but no green tea. After ten weeks, the control group had developed an average of 22.5 lung tumors per mouse. But the green tea group only developed 12.2 tumors per mouse, *a 45% reduction in cancerous tumors.*[4]

Scientists were intrigued by the results. The green tea polyphenols appeared to fight off cancer, but just what was the active ingredient? They quickly isolated five major types of polyphenols in green tea—*gallocatechin (GC), epicatechin (EC), epigallocatechin (EGC), epicatechin gallate (ECg),* and *epigallocatechin gallate (EGCg)*. But which one, or ones, was responsible for fighting off cancer?

Catechin	Percentage of Total Catechins in Tea
gallocatechin (GC)	1.6
epicatechin (EC)	6.4
epicatechin gallate (ECg)	13.6
epigallocatechin (EGC)	19.3
epigallocatechin gallate (EGCg)	59.1[5]

Repeating the NNK–green tea experiment on mice, using each catechin separately, the scientists discovered that the most powerful polyphenol, the one that reduced the greatest percentage of tumors (30%), was *epigallocatechin gallate (EGCg)*.[6] Many scientists now agree that EGCg has the highest level and broadest spectrum of cancer-fighting activity.

4. Xu, 1991.
5. Food Research Laboratories, Mitsui Norin. Co., Ltd.
6. Food Research Laboratories, Mitsui Norin Co., Ltd.

Other Antioxidants in Green Tea

The catechins are not the only antioxidants found in green tea. Like other green leafy plants, tea contains vitamins A, C, and E.

Vitamin A, found in the form of *beta carotene* in plants, protects the mucous membranes of the mouth, nose, esophagus, and lungs, which are our first line of defense against invading organisms. Countless studies have found that people consuming above-average amounts of beta carotene have below-average amounts of all kinds of cancer. The vitamin has also been shown to reverse precancerous sores in the mouth, and may guard against heart attacks and strokes by protecting against the oxidation of LDL cholesterol (the "bad" cholesterol). Beta carotene is found in yellow-orange vegetables such as apricots, sweet potatoes, cantaloupe, and carrots as well as in green leafy vegetables such as spinach and broccoli.

Vitamin C is well known for its ability to fight bacterial infections and lessen the effects of allergy-producing substances. Although Dr. Linus C. Pauling caused a great deal of controversy when he claimed that the vitamin prevented and possibly even cured cancer, laboratory studies are suggesting that he may have been right. Vitamin C not only stimulates the immune system to home in on and destroy foreign bodies, but also guards against free radical damage, enhances the effectiveness of other cancer treatments, and may actually be able to kill certain kinds of tumor cells.[7] Many studies have found that vitamin C protects against cancers of the oral cavity, esophagus, stomach, and pancreas, and there is now a good deal of evidence that it also protects against breast, rectal, cervical, and lung cancer.[8] Vitamin C helps guard against the oxidation of vitamins A and E, as well as some of the B complex vitamins, prolonging their effectiveness. It is

7. Prasad, 1980.
8. Block, 1991.

found in citrus fruits, berries, green and leafy vegetables (including green tea), tomatoes, and potatoes.

Vitamin E prevents oxygen from oxidizing and destroying fats, vitamins A and E, and the mineral selenium. (The vitamin is widely used in the food industry to protect oils from oxygen-induced rancidity.) E's ability to protect fats in the body is crucial. A cell's membrane (its protective outer covering) is made up of polyunsaturated fatty acids. If these fatty acids fall prey to free radicals (a process called *lipid peroxidation),* the cell can be entered easily. Vitamin E protects cell membranes against lipid peroxidation and also fights cancer by "quenching" singlet oxygen and boosting the activity of vitamin A. Epidemiological studies have shown that taking in adequate amounts of vitamin E can decrease the incidence of cancers of the lung, esophagus, and stomach, and possibly the bladder, colon, rectum, and prostate. A study done by the National Cancer Institute demonstrated that people taking vitamin E supplements for at least six months were able to cut their risk of oral cancer in half. And a study on chronic exposure to ozone in smog showed that vitamin E helped guard against lung damage. Good sources of vitamin E include wheat germ, soybeans, vegetable oils, broccoli, leafy greens, spinach, whole grains, and eggs.

How Do Green Tea Catechins Prevent Cancer?

There are many theories accounting for the cancer-protective effects of the catechins, but most scientists believe that they interfere with both the initiation and promotion stages of cancer:

- They lower the toxicity of certain carcinogens, thereby reducing their cancer-causing potential.
- They interfere with the binding of cancer-causing substances to the DNA of healthy cells.
- They act as antioxidants, protecting the body against free radical damage.

- They work together with antioxidants and enzymes in the small intestine, liver, and lungs to prevent tumors from starting.
- They inhibit tumor activation.

In these five ways, and possibly others, the powerful catechins in green tea work to ward off cancer. And many types of cancer fall before the catechin's ax:

- *Stomach cancer*—A case-controlled study of gastric cancer and diet in northern Kyushu, Japan, found that people who drank 10 or more cups of green tea per day had a decreased risk of gastric cancer.[9]
- *Pancreatic cancer*—Population surveys linked an increased consumption of green tea to a lower incidence of cancer of the pancreas.[10] Another study found that among those who drank 2 or more cups of green tea per day, the risk of developing pancreatic cancer was almost 60% lower than those who did not drink tea.[11]
- *Colon cancer*—A 1990 study published in the *Japanese Journal of Cancer Research* found that consumption of green tea lowered the risk of colon cancer.[12]
- *Esophageal cancer*—A population-based, case-controlled study in urban Shanghai found that drinking green tea helped protect against esophageal cancer. Among nonsmoking, non–alcohol–drinking participants who drank green tea, the males were 57% less likely and females 60% less likely to develop esophageal cancer than non–tea drinkers. (But drinking the tea while it was burning hot reduced or eliminated its protective effect.[13])
- *Liver cancer*—Giving oral EGCg to mice specially

9. Kono, 1988.
10. Goto, 1990.
11. Shibata, 1994.
12. Kato, 1990.
13. Goo, 1994.

bred to develop liver cancer reduced the number of liver tumors they developed, and sometimes prevented them altogether. And it didn't take much EGCg to protect the liver. Concentrations equivalent to those consumed daily by tea drinkers in Japan (6–8 cups) were all it took.[14]

- *Prostate cancer*—It's a sad truism that when Japanese men move to the United States, something happens that leaves them twenty times more likely to develop prostate cancer than they were at home! Some researchers have suggested that the reason may be the lack of green tea in their newly adopted diets. In a recent study, prostate cancer cells were mixed with testosterone, the hormone that makes them grow uncontrollably. But when green tea extract was added, the cells grew more slowly. The more green tea, the slower the growth.[15] That's good news, since prostate cancer is the second most common cancer in men, and virtually *all* men will develop it (to some degree) if they live long enough.

As research continues at hospitals and universities worldwide, we'll undoubtedly learn that more and more forms of cancer are swept aside or at least markedly slowed by the catechins (and possibly other substances) in green tea.

A Detailed Look at the Catechin-Cancer Battle

Let's take a closer look at each of the five ways in which green tea catechins may prevent cancer:

1. The catechins lower the toxicity of certain carcinogens, thereby reducing their cancer-causing potential.

14. Klaunig, 1992.
15. Carlin, 1996.

Consumption of foods that contain N-nitroso compounds (a group containing one nitrogen and one oxygen atom) is a major cause of stomach cancer. Suppose, for example, that you eat a hot dog or some other kind of cured, smoked meat that contains N-nitroso compounds known as *nitrites* (salts made from nitrous acid). When those nitrites mix with your gastric juices, they can be transformed into *nitrosamines,* a particularly nasty kind of carcinogen that causes stomach cancer. Scientists believe that the catechins, on the other hand, interfere with the transformation of nitrites to harmful nitrosamines. This could explain why Japanese living in the Shizuoka Prefecture, who drink green tea all day long, have low rates of gastric cancer, even though it's the leading cancer in Japan.[16]

A particularly potent member of the nitrosamine group, and a powerful inducer of stomach tumors, is *N-methyl-N'-nitrol-N-nitrosoguanidine,* or MNNG, for short. To test the catechin's prowess against carcinogens, researchers exposed various kinds of bacteria to powerful doses of MNNG. In addition to the carcinogen, some of the bacteria were also given concentrated amounts of catechins in the form of green tea extract. The bacteria that *didn't* receive the green tea extract developed 55–60% more cancerous mutations than those that did get extract.[17]

In another study using bacteria, green tea protected against the highly toxic substance aflatoxin. Aflatoxin is produced by a mold that grows on peanuts and is one of the world's most potent carcinogens. Twenty times more toxic than DDT, it has been linked to high rates of cancer, especially liver cancer,[18] as well as to mental retardation. In this study, aflatoxin and two other strong carcinogens (extracts of coal tar pitch and benzopyrene, which is found in the burned part of charbroiled foods)

16. Oguni, 1992.
17. Jain, 1989.
18. Murray, *The Healing Power of Foods,* p. 189.

were used to induce mutations in the bacteria. Half of the bacteria were given protective doses of catechins; half were not. Despite being pitted against some of the most powerful carcinogens known to man, the catechins were able to inhibit mutation in the bacteria *by more than 95%*.[19]

It certainly looked as if green tea could help prevent cancerous changes in *bacteria*. But would it prevent or slow the initiation of cancer in animals? In a study involving rats, a "test group" was given injections of a green tea extract, while a similar "control group" was not. Twenty-four hours later, both groups were injected with aflatoxin to induce cancerous changes in the bone marrow. The results? Those that received the green tea injections had considerably fewer aflatoxin-induced cancerous changes in their bone marrow cells than those who did not receive green tea.[20]

Scientists at the Skin Diseases Research Center in Cleveland, Ohio, tested green tea against several skin cancer carcinogens, using groups of hairless mice. These mice are often used in experiments because their hairless skin is very similar to that of humans, making them the next best thing to experimenting on people. In one study, half of the mice were fed green tea catechins via their drinking water for 50 days, while the other half received plain water. Then the mice were injected with potent skin cancer-causing substances (DMBA, a tumor initiator, and TPA, a promoter). At the end of the experiment, the catechin-fed group showed significantly fewer skin tumors (44% fewer) than those that did *not* receive the green tea.[21]

Then the researchers decided to find out if green tea catechins could offer any protection if they were painted on the animal's skins. Mice that were previously injected with DMBA (the cancer initiator) were divided

19. Wang, *Mutation Research,* 1989.
20. Ito, 1989.
21. Wang, *Carcinogenesis,* 1989.

into two groups—one group had a catechin solution applied topically, while the others received nothing. Just 30 minutes later, both groups were exposed to the tumor promoter, TPA. Those who had received the topical catechin application showed a reduction in skin tumor promotion of between 50 and 84%.[22]

These experiments on mouse skin were repeated but this time a different carcinogen was used—ultraviolet radiation (UVB)—rays that produce skin cancer. Those receiving catechins (either topically or through their water supply) suffered from significantly fewer sunburn lesions and skin tumors. (Topical application resulted in a 20% reduction, while ingestion resulted in a 41% reduction.)[23] And not only were there fewer UVB-induced skin tumors, those that did develop were smaller.[24]

Luckily for us, the protective effect of the catechins isn't limited just to bacteria, mice, or rats—it may also extend to humans, at least when it comes to stomach cancer. A Japanese case-controlled study on gastric cancer found that people who drank the highest amounts of green tea (10 or more cups per day) had a *40% lower* risk of developing this form of cancer than those who drank 0–4 cups per day.[25] A similar study found that the relative risk of gastric cancer was 33% less for those drinking 4 or more cups of green tea daily than for those who drank fewer.[26]

The largest population-based case-controlled study of green tea and stomach cancer was conducted in Shanghai, China. Seven hundred and eleven people with primary stomach cancer were matched with 711 controls who lived in the same area, were of the same age and gender, but did not have the cancer. This study revealed that those who drank green tea habitually—

22. Mukhtar, 1992.
23. Mukhtar, 1992.
24. Ibid, and Conney, 1992.
25. Kono, 1988.
26. Tajima, 1985.

one cup of green tea or more per week for the past six months—had a 29% lower risk of stomach cancer than those who didn't. Interestingly, it didn't seem to matter how old the person was when he or she began to drink green tea habitually.[27] Even late starters were protected, which suggests that it's never too late to begin sipping green tea. (Some laboratory experiments, however, suggest that the earlier the exposure to polyphenols, the better. The offspring of rats that were fed catechins while pregnant, for example, were found to be far more resistant to breast cancer development than the offspring of other rats.[28])

2. *The catechins interfere with the binding of cancer-causing substances to the DNA of healthy cells.*

Once a carcinogen binds with the DNA, it "hijacks" the cell and begins issuing orders on its own. The cell's structure and function are then altered as it is initiated into its new life as a cancer cell. But if the offending substance could be prevented from binding to the cell's DNA in the first place, the cancer process would never take place. And catechins appear to do just that.

The mice mentioned earlier that were "painted" with a catechin solution and thereby developed fewer tumors were able to resist the cancer process for one big reason: The catechins prevented the carcinogen from binding to the DNA in the epidermal cells.[29]

Other studies have also shown the catechin's inhibition of the binding process. When rats were fed a powder made from green tea, the binding ability of DMBA (a carcinogen responsible for breast cancer) fell by 75%.[30] And the binding of the carcinogen benzopyrene to calf thymus DNA was also found to be significantly inhibited by four different catechins (EC, EGC, ECg, and EGCg).[31]

27. Yu, 1995.
28. Food Research Laboratories, Mitsui Norin Co., Ltd.
29. Mukhtar, 1992.
30. Sakamoto, 1994.
31. Ibid.

If the carcinogen can't stick, it can't make you sick. And the catechins prevent the sticking.

3. *The catechins act as antioxidants, protecting the body against free radical damage.*

Green tea contains a broad array of antioxidants (including the catechins, vitamin C, vitamin E, and the bioflavonoids) that trap and destroy free radicals. These antioxidants also interfere with free radical chain reactions, preventing damage to the body's cells and tissues.[32]

Green tea's main ingredient in the fight against free radicals is EGCg.[33] Among other things, EGCg extends its strongly protective umbrella over the fatty acids and lipids in the brain. These fatty acids and lipids are particularly susceptible to the effects of free radical *peroxidation,* a process like that of the cooking oil in your kitchen turning rancid. (Peroxidation is believed to be responsible for much of the aging of the brain.) By keeping these parts of the brain "fresh," EGCg helps to keep us young, alert, and able.

Preservatives such as vitamin E or BHA are often added to cooking oil to keep it from going rancid. But in laboratory tests using salad oil, *green tea catechins showed much stronger antioxidant effects than either vitamin E or BHA,*[34] and when combined with vitamins E and/or C, the catechins' effects were even more pronounced.[35] In a similar finding, researchers reported in *Cell Biophysics* that green tea was a more effective free radical scavenger than either vitamin C or vitamin E.[36]

And through their antioxidative action, the catechins are even able to fight a deadly carcinogen found in cigarette smoke. When rats were given green tea and then exposed to NNK, one of cigarette smoke's most potent cancer-causing components, the catechins inhib-

32. Yang, 1993.
33. Ho, 1992.
34. Matsuzaki, 1985.
35. Food Research Laboratories, Mitsui Norin Co., Ltd.
36. Zhao, 1989.

ited "single-strand breaks" in the DNA of the rats' liver cells.[37] This is important because any damage to the DNA can start the cancer process rolling, so by preventing this first, disabling blow, carcinogenesis may be avoided altogether.

Stopping the Killer Before It Starts

"EGCg may prevent the activation of certain carcinogens so that the free radicals never form."
—Fung-Lung Chung, Chemist,
American Health Foundation

---

4. The catechins work together with antioxidants and enzymes in the small intestine, liver, and lungs to prevent tumors from starting.

Besides acting as antioxidants themselves, the catechins work in tandem with the other antioxidants, increasing their protective effects on the body's healthy cells. They help to strengthen the capillary blood vessels, guard against damage to cell membranes, and decrease the rate of oxidation of fats (a known cause of cancer).

A 1992 study reported in the journal *Cancer Research* confirms the idea that green tea can "rev up" certain enzymes and antioxidants in the body. After feeding catechins to hairless mice for thirty days, scientists found that the activities of both antioxidants and good enzymes in the small bowel, liver, and lungs had increased.[38] Researchers at the American Health Foundation in Valhalla, New York, also reported that catechins had a helpful effect on enzymes in the human liver. The ability of two liver enzymes (cytochrome P450 and glucuronyltransferase) to neutralize and excrete

37. Liu, 1991.
38. Kahn, 1992.

toxic substances increased when subjects were given green tea catechins.[39]

5. *The catechins inhibit tumor activation.*

Earlier we noted that hairless mice injected with carcinogens didn't develop as many tumors because green tea catechins were put in their drinking water or were painted on their skins. Other studies have also confirmed the ability of catechins to inhibit tumor activation. Researchers at the Laboratory for Cancer Research at Rutgers University in New Jersey found that giving green tea orally inhibited the formation of tumors in the forestomach and lung in mice already initiated with carcinogens. Any tumors that did form were markedly smaller.[40] And researchers at the National Cancer Center Research Institute in Tokyo, Japan, found that green tea (specifically EGCg) inhibited tumor promotion in both the skin and gastrointestinal tract of mice. Their conclusion: EGCg "is a practical cancer chemopreventive agent available in everyday life."[41]

In recent studies, the catechins have been shown to block tumor formation in the liver,[42] esophagus,[43] skin,[44] lung, forestomach, small intestine, colon, liver, pancreas, and mammary gland.[45] And catechins have even slowed the growth of tumors that are already established. In ten different experiments, mice that had skin tumors were given either green tea extracts in their drinking water or injections of EGCg three times a week for 4–10 weeks. In five of these studies, tumor growth was inhibited by *up to 90%,* with the other five experiments showing "marked inhibition of tumor growth" (46–89%). Complete tumor regression occurred in 4%

39. Weisburger, 1991.
40. Conney, 1992.
41. Fujiki, 1992.
42. Klaunig, 1992.
43. Chen, 1992.
44. Fujiki, 1992.
45. Blot, 1993.

of the mice treated with green tea—compared to no regression at all in those who did not receive green tea.[46]

To Your Health!

"Current research shows that tea contains powerful antioxidants and health promoting ingredients, lowering the risk of heart disease and certain types of cancer. Thus, hot or iced tea intake to fill the daily liquid requirements can contribute to good health."
—John Weisburger, Ph.D.,
American Health Foundation

Extending Life?

There is no cure for cancer, but scientifically valid studies conducted by respected scientists the world over have shown that green tea is a powerful weapon against this devastating and deadly affliction. Perhaps Eisai was right when he wrote, back in A.D. 1211: "Tea is a miraculous medicine for the maintenance of health. Tea has an extraordinary power to prolong life." By warding off the number two killer disease in America, green tea can greatly increase our chances of living long and healthy lives.

---

46. Wang, *Cancer Research*, March 1, 1992.

CHAPTER 4

Getting to the Heart of the Matter

Tea is used all over the Indies, not only among those of the country, but also among the Dutch and the English, who take it as a drug.
— JOHN ALBRECHT VON MANDELSLO, 1662, *Travels into the East Indies*

College basketball star Hank Gathers suddenly crumpled to the floor in the middle of a game. He was carried off on a stretcher and died shortly thereafter at the age of twenty-two. Olympic gold medal–winning skater Sergei Grinkov collapsed during practice, never again to regain consciousness. Entertainer Tiny Tim keeled over after performing at a benefit and died in a nearby hospital. The same, sneaky culprit—heart disease—was responsible for each of these tragedies, and these victims certainly don't stand alone. About 500,000 people die of heart disease each year in the United States, making it our number one killer disease. And eventually it will cause the deaths of *about half of all Americans living today*.

It's terrifying to think that your heart, that all-important fuel pump, can suddenly stop working. Unfortunately, it happens every day. One and a half million Americans will suffer heart attacks this year and more than 6 million living Americans have experienced heart attacks or chest pain (angina pectoris) or both.

Since the odds are so high that we'll fall prey to this killer disease, we owe it to ourselves and our families to do whatever we can to lower our risk. Many factors contribute to the development of heart disease, and it's vitally important to keep them in check. They include high blood cholesterol levels, high blood pressure, cigarette smoking, high blood fats, obesity, high stress levels, lack of exercise, and diabetes mellitus. The surprising news is that (with the exception of lack of exercise) *drinking green tea can help mediate all of these factors*. This doesn't mean that just because you drink green tea you can gobble all of the high-fat, high-cholesterol foods that you want without affecting your cardiovascular system, but it can serve as an excellent adjunct to your other heart-healthy habits. Before we find out how, let's take a quick look at the heart.

The Wonder Pump—and the Attacks It Suffers

The heart is the body's fuel pump, servicing every single cell with some 100,000 deliveries of oxygen and nutrients per day via the bloodstream. The heart pumps an average of 60–100 times per minute and, over a lifetime, beats as many as 3 billion times! The heart automatically adjusts the speed of its beats according to the body's immediate needs. Under stress, during heavy exercise, or when engaging in enthusiastic sex, the heart may pump as many as 170 times a minute, but during sleep it may cut way back to only 50 or 60 times a minute. Throughout a lifetime, this hard-working muscle never stops to rest except between beats, and in the average person continues plodding along for some seventy-seven years.

Most of what we call "heart disease" is really *coronary artery disease (CAD)*. Like all body tissue, the hard-working heart muscle must receive a continual supply of oxygen and nutrients from the blood. The heart gets its blood via the *coronary arteries,* blood vessels that sit atop the heart muscle and look something like a crown. (*Corona* means "crown.") These arteries are tiny compared to some found in the body, and it doesn't take much to plug them up. If and when that happens, you've got a big problem. Once a coronary artery becomes clogged, heart tissue "downstream" of the blockage dies. This death of the heart tissue due to a lack of blood is commonly referred to as a *heart attack.*

Clogged arteries are a major cause of heart attacks, and the most common artery clogger is *plaque,* a fatty substance made up of cholesterol, fat, blood clots, and/or cellular debris. Plaque accumulates on artery walls the way rust accumulates inside old pipes, growing thicker and thicker until finally the tube is completely blocked and nothing can pass through. When plaque builds up inside your arteries it causes a condition called *atherosclerosis,* which is a major risk factor for heart disease. Besides triggering a heart attack, atherosclerosis can also lead to a stroke, if the artery that becomes blocked happens to supply blood to the brain.

The gradual clogging of arteries isn't the only way that plaque can trigger a heart attack or stroke. More commonly, people get into trouble when a little piece of plaque breaks off from an artery wall and begins to float through the bloodstream. This free-floating plaque is something like a little rubber ball floating through your home's plumbing system. The ball will slide easily through some of the pipes, but somewhere along the line it will find itself inside a pipe that's too narrow to let it pass. Lodged in place, the ball will block the flow of water, and anything downstream of the blockage will simply dry up. The same thing happens to a piece of plaque floating along in your arteries. It passes easily through larger arteries, but sooner or later it gets stuck and blocks up a smaller one. Anything downstream then "dries up" (and in this case, dies) from a lack of fresh blood.

Many factors contribute to the formation of arterial plaque, including dietary fat, smoking, and heredity, but more often than not, the villain is excess *cholesterol* in the blood.

Cholesterol and Heart Disease

Cholesterol is a waxy, fatty substance that is manufactured in the liver and found in all animal tissues. It's used in many different ways in the body: to build cell membranes, as an insulating sheath around nerve fibers, and as a basis for certain hormones, just to name a few. We need a certain amount of cholesterol. The problems begin when we have too much of it.

Blood cholesterol is measured by taking a sample of your blood and analyzing it. Your cholesterol level (referred to as your *total cholesterol)* is expressed as milligrams per deciliter (mg/dl) or the number of milligrams of cholesterol per tenth of a liter (deciliter) of your blood. Anything under 200 mg/dl is considered normal, between 201 and 240 is considered borderline, and over 240 is considered high.

There are two other important cholesterol levels: the *HDL (high-density lipoproteins)* and the *LDL (low-density lipoproteins)*. Cholesterol cannot travel around the body unaided—it needs to "hitch a ride" on something else. By hooking up with protein and fat (thus forming a *lipoprotein)*, cholesterol is able to circulate throughout the bloodstream. HDL and LDL are two different kinds of lipoproteins with one big difference to your health: HDL carries cholesterol *away* from artery walls, while LDL carries cholesterol *to* them.

The Good, the Bad, and the Ugly

HDL (often called the "good cholesterol") picks up excess cholesterol and brings it back to the liver for excretion or reprocessing. But the *LDL* (the "bad cholesterol") continues to circulate through the bloodstream, eventually depositing its cholesterol on arterial walls. So if your HDL levels are low, or your LDL levels are high, you're more likely to develop arterial deposits (plaque). Here's how to interpret your HDL and LDL test results:

	HDL	LDL
Desirable	Over 65	Under 130
Borderline	35–64	130–159
At Risk	34 or less	160 or more

Studies have shown that HDL levels of 70 or more can protect against heart disease, while those that are below 35 can indicate coronary risk. LDL levels under 130 are considered desirable, between 130–159 are considered borderline, and 160 or above are considered high. In order to get a true picture of your coronary risk, though, all three cholesterol levels (total cholesterol, HDL, and LDL) must be taken into account. You may think that you're home free because your total cholesterol level is low, but if your LDL is high or your HDL is low, you may be still at risk for heart disease.

Sipping Away the Risk of Heart Disease

Whether your risk is high or low, whether you're in good health or poor, you'd probably like to ensure that your heart and cardiovascular system stay healthy. There are many ways to do this, but one that's simple, convenient, and always satisfying is as near as your friendly teapot—drinking a nice, hot cup of green tea! In study after study, green tea has been found to lower cholesterol levels, stop the platelets from forming deadly clots, fight free radicals that encourage arterial buildup, lower high blood pressure, fight heart-straining obesity, and reduce stress. Even the most expensive medicine in the world can't claim to provide all these cardioprotective effects—but green tea does, and for just pennies a cup.

So let's take a look at the many ways this time-tested beverage works its heart-protecting miracles.

Tea Drinking Lowers Cholesterol Levels

Studies showing that drinking tea can lower blood cholesterol levels have been performed in laboratories around the world. For example:

- A Japanese study of 1,306 men found that those who drank 9 or more cups of green tea daily had cholesterol levels that were an average of 8 mg/dl lower than those who drank 0–2 cups of tea per day.[1] This 8-point drop is significant, for it's been estimated that for every 1 percent drop in cholesterol, there is a 2 percent reduction in heart disease risk. That means that the subjects of this Japanese study were 16 percent less likely to develop heart disease than their non–tea-drinking counterparts.
- Scientists in Norway studying 9,857 men found that the greater the consumption of black tea, the lower the levels of both total cholesterol and systolic blood pressure (the first number in a blood pressure reading). And during a twelve-year follow-up period, those who drank one or more cups of tea per day had a *lower mortality rate* than those who drank no tea.[2]
- In Israel, researchers also found that drinkers of black tea had lower cholesterol levels, while coffee drinkers had both higher total cholesterol and "bad" LDL cholesterol levels. In addition, they noted that tea drinkers tended to have fewer negative health-related habits (such as smoking and drinking alcoholic beverages) than coffee drinkers.[3]

1. Kono, *Preventive Medicine,* 1992.
2. Stensvold, 1992.
3. Green, 1992.

This last bit of information made the scientists stop and think. Was it the *tea* that was responsible for the lower cholesterol levels, or was it the *lifestyle* of the typical tea drinker? Perhaps people who drank tea took better care of themselves, smoked less, or ate a lower-fat diet. Indeed, one study of 20,000 people found that the more tea that women drank, the fewer cookies they consumed (although the opposite appeared to be true for men). In addition, it was found that both male and female tea drinkers ate more bread, took more vitamins and/or cod liver oil, ate more oranges, drank less coffee, and smoked fewer cigarettes than those who drank no tea.[4]

But even after adjusting for smoking, alcohol use, physical activity, and body mass index, researchers in Japan found that cholesterol levels were inversely related to the consumption of green tea—that is, the more green tea people consumed, the lower their cholesterol levels.[5]

And green tea's beneficial effects are not just limited to driving down the total cholesterol and the "bad" LDL cholesterol. A study of 1,371 men in Yoshimi, Japan, found that increased consumption of green tea (especially more than 10 cups per day) was associated with lower blood fat (triglyceride) levels and a lessened tendency toward atherosclerosis. (As a side benefit, the green tea also offered some protection against damage to liver cells.)[6]

Green tea was clearly helpful in the battle against elevated cholesterol, but would it still be useful if people ate the worst kind of diet? Scientists at the Food Research Laboratories of Mitsui Norin Company in Japan decided to find out. Knowing that excess saturated fat raises blood cholesterol levels, the researchers fed rats diets rich in lard and cholesterol to induce elevated blood cholesterol levels. Half of the rats were also given

4. Stensvold, 1992.
5. Kono, *Preventive Medicine*, 1992.
6. Imai, 1995.

a powdered form of green tea (the human equivalent of about 20 cups of tea per day).

The results? The animals that *did not* receive the green tea wound up with cholesterol levels *twice as high* as those that did. In addition, harmful LDL increased up to *fifteen times* in response to the lard-cholesterol diet, while their beneficial HDL was cut to less than half. Cholesterol levels in the green tea group also rose on the lard-cholesterol diet, but the increase was only about half as high as in the control group, and the fall in HDL levels was not as severe.[7] Clearly, the green tea exerted a protective effect against serious heart disease risk factors, even when the most heart-clogging kind of diet was consumed.

But how, exactly, does green tea lower blood cholesterol? Scientists at the Kyoto Pharmaceutical University in Japan reported that green tea helped to suppress the absorption of cholesterol in the digestive tracts of rats, while increasing excretion of excess cholesterol.[8] Muramatsu et al. also noted increased fecal excretion of fat and cholesterol in rats receiving the green tea catechins.[9] In other words, green tea encourages the body to absorb less cholesterol while excreting more, resulting in lower total cholesterol levels.

Green Tea Eliminates Dangerous "Stickiness"

One theory explaining the origins of coronary artery disease is that it begins with an injury to the wall of a vein or artery (and it may be a very small injury). As part of the healing process, platelets (the smallest cells in the blood) release a substance called *thromboxane*, which causes the platelets to clump together to form a plug *(thrombus)*. Once the plug attaches to the wall of the vein or artery, it protrudes into the bloodstream,

7. Hara, 1991.
8. Chisaka, 1988.
9. Muramatsu, 1986.

obstructing the flow of blood to some degree. Cholesterol, blood fats, and cellular debris then become caught on this plug, slowly forming a dam that eventually stops the blood flow entirely. Another scenario: An injury occurs, the plug forms and then breaks loose from the vessel wall, floating through the circulatory system (like a piece of plaque) until it finds itself stuck in a narrow blood vessel, where it blocks the flow of blood. But to make matters worse, the substance that causes the platelets to clump together in the first place *(thromboxane)* also causes blood vessels to *constrict,* making their passageways even smaller.

While we need a certain amount of platelet aggregation to ensure that we don't bleed to death when we cut ourselves, we don't want those cells to stick together too much. For years doctors have treated sticky platelet conditions with "blood thinners" such as aspirin, coumarin, or warfarin. But these, like all drugs, have potentially dangerous side effects like gastrointestinal problems and skin rashes. What we really needed was something that could keep our platelets from becoming too sticky without walloping us with side effects.

Green tea is that elusive "something" we've been looking for. In tests on platelet aggregation in rabbits, researchers discovered that hot water extract of green tea *inhibited the formation of clots as effectively as aspirin,* the most widely used, well-known blood thinner in existence. Upon further examination, scientists discovered that the substance in green tea mainly responsible for this anticlotting effect was EGCg.[10]

These results were confirmed by researchers at Zhejing Medical University Hospital in China, who found that tea helped to reduce blood coagulation, prevent platelet stickiness and clumping, decrease the amount of cholesterol in the artery walls, and even help *break down clots that had already formed.*[11]

10. Sagesaka-Mitane, 1990.
11. Lou, 1991.

Green tea's ability to protect against strokes, many of which are caused by blocked arteries in the brain, was borne out in epidemiological studies. Researchers looking at 6,000 Japanese subjects age forty or older discovered that the more green tea the people drank, the lower their chances of having a stroke. While 2% of those who drank no green tea had strokes or a history of stroke, only 0.4% of those who drank 3–4 cups per day had strokes or stroke history. During a 4-year follow-up period, those who drank more than 5 cups of green tea daily had *less than half the incidence of stroke and cerebral hemorrhage* than those who drank less.[12]

But how did green tea keep the deadly clots from forming, thereby lowering the chance of heart attacks and strokes? In 1990, scientists finally figured out that green tea's EGCg was able to inhibit the action of thromboxane, the substance responsible for both clot formation and blood vessel constriction.[13] When the action of thromboxane was inhibited, blood vessels remained wide open, fewer clots formed, and those that did form were more easily broken down. For years doctors had prescribed thromboxane inhibitors to relax the blood vessels and guard against clots. Little did they know that a completely natural substance with no side effects (except health-boosting ones!) could do the same thing.

Green Tea Guards Against Free Radical Damage

Earlier we said that an injury to the artery wall begins the process of plaque buildup by forming an obstruction in the bloodstream. Now scientists believe that fat and cholesterol in the blood (especially LDL) can actually be the *cause* of that injury.[14] LDL, as you know, likes to hang out on arterial walls. When it's attacked by free radicals (oxidized), LDL becomes irritating to the artery

12. Sato, 1989.
13. Ali, 1990.
14. Perdue, p. 204.

wall and can actually "wound" it. Or it's possible that oxidized LDL traveling through the bloodstream is more likely to be deposited at the site of an existing wound. Either way, free radicals play an important part in encouraging the formation of excess plaque on artery walls.[15]

We know that green tea contains powerful antioxidants that can guard the skin against UVB radiation, stimulate liver enzymes to deactivate toxins, and protect fats and oils from rancidity. It makes sense, then, that green tea should offer some protection against the free radicals implicated in coronary artery disease.

LDL is most vulnerable to oxidation when floating through the blood that has just come from the lungs and is full of oxygen. The newly oxygenated blood gets its final send-off from the heart and is sent surging through the aorta on its way to the rest of the body. For reasons yet unknown, it's at this point that the LDL "sheds" the antioxidants that normally travel with it. Exposed to massive amounts of oxygen, the LDL can easily be attacked by free radicals. Luckily, high-quality antioxidants such as those found in green tea also make their way through the bloodstream, binding with the LDL cholesterol and "standing in" for the antioxidants that were lost in the aorta. Studies conducted at the University of Scranton in Pennsylvania showed that because they were superior sources of antioxidants, both black and green teas were very effective at preventing the oxidation of LDL and the subsequent clogging of the blood vessels.[16]

So green tea can lower cholesterol, keep platelets from clumping together, and knock out the free radical action that sets atherosclerosis in motion. These three accomplishments alone should get it nominated as the "Heart Protective Medicine of the Year." But it can do even more.

15. Fox, B., *Foods to Heal By*, p. 12.
16. Tufts University Diet & Nutrition Letter.

Green Tea Helps Keep Blood Pressure Under Control

High blood pressure (also known as hypertension) is one of the most important warning signs of heart disease. It's called "the silent killer" because you can't feel it. But just the same, over time it can wreak havoc on your cardiovascular system. Just as too much water pressure can cause water pipes to crack, too much blood pressure can cause small cracks to form in artery walls. These cracks are ideal places for clots and plaque to form, and before you know it, you have the markings of a heart attack or stroke. Additionally, the heart may have to work so hard to force the blood through partially clogged blood vessels that it becomes enlarged and eventually just gives out.

Normal arteries are wide open, flexible tubes that stretch and relax as the blood surges through, responding to the ebb and flow. But if the heart should start to beat harder and faster, or if the arteries narrow, the blood pressure will go up.

Many factors can cause arteries to narrow—plaque buildup, smoking, poor diet, genetic factors, alcoholism, stress, lack of exercise, certain diseases such as diabetes, or a "signal" from the body. This "signal" is the release of an enzyme called ACE (angiotensin converting enzyme). ACE starts a chain reaction that causes the tiny muscles surrounding the arteries to clamp down, making the arteries smaller and driving up blood pressure. Preventing this "clamping down" of the muscles and keeping the arteries from narrowing is an important step in preventing high blood pressure. There are several antihypertensive drugs on the market that work by blocking the action of ACE, but like the thromboxane inhibitors, they have side effects—in this case, loss of taste, diarrhea, and possible swelling of the mouth, face, and hands.

Fortunately, we don't have to rely on drugs to protect

us from high blood pressure. Green tea also inhibits ACE and lowers blood pressure, without the nasty side effects. To test the effects of green tea on hypertension, mice that were specially bred to have high blood pressure were divided into two groups, just one week after they were weaned. One group received a normal diet, while the other was given the same diet plus 0.5% crude catechins. At ten weeks of age, the blood pressures of the mice with the normal diet had already skyrocketed, while those of the catechin-fed mice were significantly lower. Then, at sixteen weeks of age, the diets of the two groups were switched. Within three weeks, the mice now receiving catechins (whose blood pressures had formerly gone through the roof) had lower blood pressures than the other group.[17]

In another study, green tea was found to prolong significantly the life spans of stroke-prone rats that had high blood pressure. Once again, one group was given a normal diet, while the other group was given the same diet plus 0.5% crude catechins. The rats receiving the catechins lived an average of 27% longer than those who didn't receive them, prompting the researchers to conclude that "a daily intake of tea polyphenols could prevent or delay the occurrence of cardiovascular diseases."[18]

Carrying it one step further, researchers gave 500 mg doses of green tea catechins to 37 human volunteers with high blood pressure, high blood sugar, and high serum cholesterol. The volunteers took the catechins after breakfast and after lunch every day for at least twelve weeks. At the end of the study, researchers found that the tea catechins had significantly lowered blood pressure and triglyceride levels, while raising the "good" HDL.[19]

17. Hara, 1991.
18. Ibid.
19. Kanaya.

Green tea is clearly an effective aid in the battle against high blood pressure, but the "miracle" doesn't end here.

Green Tea and Diabetes

Diabetes, a condition characterized by an excess of glucose in the bloodstream, is a devastating disease that attacks virtually every part of the body. Glucose (often referred to as "blood sugar") is the body's fuel. It travels through the bloodstream searching for hungry cells in need of energy. But once the glucose arrives at a hungry cell, it can't just "walk in" to the cell; it needs the help of the hormone called *insulin*. The insulin acts like a key that fits into a lock called the *insulin receptor site*. When insulin "turns the key," glucose can enter the cell.

When people have diabetes, either they're not making enough insulin to get the glucose into the cells, or the insulin fails to "unlock" the cell and let the sugar enter. Why wouldn't the insulin be able to "unlock" the cell? The most common culprit is obesity. When too many fat cells crowd in next to other cells, they can block the area where the insulin "key" is supposed to fit. Then the "key" can't get to the lock, so even if plenty of glucose is available, the cell can't get it. It's as if a thick, juicy steak has been presented to a person whose jaw is wired shut. No matter how ravenous the person may be, there is no way in the world that person could eat that steak. A similar situation occurs when insufficient amounts of insulin are produced. There's just not enough fuel making it into the tank.

In either case, glucose that can't get into the cell continues to sail downstream, leaving the cell starved for energy. Realizing that its cells are still hungry, the body pushes more and more glucose into the bloodstream. Blood sugar levels rise dramatically, but the sugar still doesn't get into the cells. Instead, its high levels in the blood ravage the body. Long-term damage can be severe, including such devastating effects as gangrene (especially of the feet), ulcers, kidney failure, and blindness. Diabetes is also a major risk factor for heart disease and stroke because it makes the blood vessels less elastic and more likely to become clogged with plaque.

How can drinking green tea help control an all-consuming disease like diabetes? By going right to the source of the problem—the formation of blood glucose. Glucose is one of the building blocks of complex carbohydrates (better known as starches) found in foods. The starch molecule is like a string of pearls, with each pearl representing a molecule of glucose. Your body can't absorb the starch molecule as a whole—it has to be broken apart. A special enzyme called *amylase* does just that, acting like a pair of scissors to cut each pearl loose from the string. These single pearls, or glucose molecules, are then able to be absorbed into the bloodstream and used as fuel.

But green tea polyphenols have been found to be potent *inhibitors* of amylase. It's as if green tea dulls the enzyme's cutting power and "rusts" its scissors-like effect until it's almost worthless. In fact, in laboratory tests the amount of polyphenols in just *one cup of green tea* was found to inhibit 87% of amylase's activity.[20] And if less sugar gets into the bloodstream, blood glucose levels will automatically be lowered.

Nice theory, but does it work? Well, scientists seem to think so. One study found that feeding tea catechins to rats reduced both blood glucose and insulin levels,[21] and that catechins were very effective starch and sucrose blockers in the digestive tracts of rats.[22] Happily, similar results were observed in humans. When 300 mg of tea catechins were given to subjects ten minutes before tak-

20. Hara, 1990.
21. Matsumoto, 1993.
22. Hara, 1990.

ing in 50 g of starch, their glucose and insulin levels did not rise nearly as much as was expected.[23]

Besides its starch-blocking effect, green tea may also help get rid of excess fat, the villain that can cause diabetes or make it much worse. That's great news for diabetics—and for many of the rest of us, too.

Staying Slim with Green Tea

The link between obesity and coronary artery disease has been well established for years. A person whose body weight is more than 20% greater than ideal often has high cholesterol, high blood fat levels, and an over-worked heart. High blood pressure runs rampant among overweight people, especially those between the ages of twenty and forty-five, who are 5.6 times more likely to be hypertensive than their slim counterparts.[24]

Obese women seem to be particularly hard-hit by heart disease. Researchers at Harvard Medical School studied 115,000 women aged thirty to fifty-five for eight years and found that 40 percent of those who developed heart disease had no risk factors for heart disease *except* being overweight.[25]

Obesity can also contribute to diabetes, which is three times more likely to occur in overweight people than in those of normal weight.[26] The accumulation of fat cells around the insulin receptor sites makes it impossible for insulin to "unlock" the cell, so glucose can't enter. Blood sugar rises and bodily damage ensues. But once the excess weight is lost, the receptor sites become unblocked and insulin can get in to do its job. Prevention of obesity, then, is a critical factor in treating diabetes.

Whoever discovers the "cure" for obesity will most

23. Food Research Laboratories, 1993.
24. The Wellness Encyclopedia, pp. 22–23.
25. Ibid.
26. Fox, A., 1996, p. 263.

certainly win the Nobel Prize. Green tea cannot claim to be that cure, but it has shown some promising effects in preliminary tests. Consider the following:

When rats were fed catechins along with a normal diet, their accumulation of body fat dropped. In fact, after one month, rats fed a diet containing 5% catechins had an average body fat of 7%, while rats fed the same diet without the catechins had an average 11% body fat. Reduction in body fat continued in the catechin-fed group for about three months, after which it leveled off, thereby confirming the catechins' safety.[27] (In other words, green tea catechins will automatically stop reducing body fat at a certain point. You won't lose too much weight.)

In another study, rats were fed a diet containing 15% palm oil, a highly saturated fat guaranteed to make them accumulate excess body and liver fat. One group received the palm oil diet, a second group received the palm oil diet plus 1% catechins, and a third group ate a normal diet. The group that got the palm oil diet gained excess body and liver fat, but in the catechin-fed group *this gain was suppressed. In fact, the catechin-fed group had body and liver fat levels almost comparable to those consuming a normal diet!*[28] This suggests that it may be possible for green tea to control obesity even if you are eating a poor diet! (Note: A 5% catechin diet is the equivalent of about 20 cups of tea per day for humans.)

Relieving Stress with Green Tea

Stress can be defined as emotional, physical, and/or mental anguish arising from the demands of everyday life. When a steam engine is overloaded, steam rushes out the escape valve, but unfortunately we humans don't have an escape valve. Over time, stress can take a terrible

27. Food Research Laboratories.
28. Food Research Laboratories, 1993.

physical toll, especially on the heart. In fact, it's been estimated that nearly 80% of all coronary artery disease is associated with stress.[29]

How does stress prompt CAD? By flooding the body with high-voltage chemicals such as adrenaline, nor-adrenalin, and ACTH that cause the blood pressure to rise, the blood fats, cholesterol, and blood sugar to increase, and the arteries to constrict. Even the coronary arteries clamp down in response to stress, restricting the flow of blood to the heart muscle itself.

The deleterious effects of stress to the heart were documented in a study published in the *Journal of the American Medical Association* in June 1996.[30] Researchers studied 112 men and 14 women suffering from coronary artery disease. When some of these people were mentally stressed, the flow of blood to their hearts dropped. Of the group, these people were found to be significantly more likely to suffer from fatal and nonfatal heart attacks.

Scientists have not yet studied the effects of green tea on stress, but it makes sense that stopping for a cup of tea and temporarily throwing aside the cares of the day should help counteract tension and anxiety. The Japanese have elevated the drinking of tea to an art form with their tea ceremony, or *Cha-no-yu*. (*See* Chapter 8 for a complete description.) Held in the open air or a simple tea room, the ceremony revolves around simplicity, cleanliness, serenity, and grace. Meditation also plays an important role in the tea ceremony. The Japanese believe that although it is impossible to live a life completely free of stress, it is always possible to have less stress.

The health benefits of the tea ceremony were scientifically documented in 1992 in a study of more than 3,000 women aged fifty or older living in Tokyo. Those

29. The United States Clearing House for Mental Health Information.
30. Wei, 1996.

that practiced the tea ceremony regularly were found to live longer than the average Tokyo woman.[31]

But even those who do not practice *Cha-no-yu* can find relief from stress in a cup of tea. It is one of life's simple pleasures, a chance to sit down, relax, chat with a friend, or just daydream. As Henry James put it so aptly in *The Portrait of a Lady*, "There are few hours in life more agreeable than the hour dedicated to the ceremony known as afternoon tea." Enjoy yourself—you (and your heart) deserve it.

A Tasty Medicine

The evidence is clear. Green tea guards against heart disease by helping to keep cholesterol and LDL down, while keeping the helpful HDL up; by preventing "sticky" platelets from damaging arteries; by protecting the heart from damaging free radicals; by pulling blood pressure down to safe levels; by reducing diabetic damage to the arteries; and by combating stress. More than simply a tasty, soothing beverage, green tea is a powerful ally in our constant struggle to defeat America's number one killer disease.

31. Sadakata, 1992.

CHAPTER 5

What Else Can Green Tea Do?

For tea, though ridiculed by those who are naturally coarse in their nervous sensibilities, or are become so from wine-drinking, and are not susceptible of influence from so refined a stimulant, will always be the favoured beverage of the intellectual . . .
— Thomas De Quincey,
Confessions of an English Opium-Eater

We've praised the ability of green tea to fight cancer and protect against heart disease and stroke—calling its effects nothing short of miraculous. But wait until you see what else it can do! Unbelievable as it may seem, this incredible substance can:

- *Fight deadly bacteria*—including those that cause cholera, pneumonia, abscesses, botulism, dysentery, and food poisoning, all without disturbing the ''friendly'' intestinal bacteria.
- *Combat oral bacteria that cause dental cavities and bad breath*—while inhibiting plaque formation and hardening tooth enamel. Even bacteria from infected root canals fall before the onslaughts of green tea!
- *Inhibit the action of viruses*—including flu virus, herpes simplex, vaccinia, Coxsackie virus B6, polio, and even part of the HIV virus by preventing its attachment to healthy cells.

- *Stimulate the immune system*—encouraging the fight against foreign invaders.
- *Prevent post-traumatic epileptic seizures* in laboratory rats.
- *Fight MRSA,* a strain of staphylococcus aureus that is resistant to drugs.
- *Slow the aging process*—by inhibiting free radical damage to cells.
- *Provide a stimulating pick-me-up*—without triggering nervousness or sleepless nights.
- *Preserve the freshness of foods and cosmetics*—working as well or better than vitamin E and/or certain chemicals such as BHA.
- *Inhibit the accumulation of excess body fat.*
- *Help suppress the appetite.*
- *Help maintain the body's fluid balance.*

Green Tea, Bacteria, and the Digestive System

Back in the 1800s, a Hungarian obstetrician named Ignaz Semmelweiss caused an uproar when he insisted that the doctors who had just finished dissecting corpses wash their hands before examining pregnant women. The doctors were somehow passing disease from the deceased to the pregnant women by way of their hands, Semmelweiss argued, and hand washing was the only way to stop it. Despite proving that hand washing prevented much of the deadly puerperal fever that was killing the pregnant women, Semmelweiss was hounded out of the profession by his fellow physicians, and eventually ended his life in an insane asylum.

Today we know that Dr. Semmelweiss was right. Bacteria and viruses are invisible to the naked eye but are virtually everywhere, not just on corpses. Although many of these small one-celled organisms are harmless, some can cause raging infections that can kill a person in a matter of days. Bacteria can be transmitted in many ways—some by way of unwashed hands, others through spoiled food, exchange of bodily fluids, touching a contaminated surface, or through a cough or a sneeze. The immune system is supposed to destroy harmful bacteria, or at least keep them under control. Sometimes, however, the immune system is too overworked to do so, or is simply unable to manage even when operating at full strength.

Fortunately, tea leaves act as an antibacterial agent, slowing or stopping the action of bacteria that cause certain dangerous and deadly diseases. Scientists at the Showa University School of Medicine in Tokyo found that tea catechins protected against infection by *Vibrio cholerae*,[1] the bacteria that causes cholera, a severe infection of the small intestine in humans and animals. In other laboratory tests, tea polyphenols inhibited not only *Vibrio cholerae,* but also *staphylococcus aureus* (a bacteria found on the skin and in the throat that causes pneumonia, abscesses, and other infections) and the deadly *Clostridium botulinum*,[2] which causes botulism.

C. botulinum belongs to the Clostridium species, a particularly toxic family of bacteria that, besides botulism, can cause gangrene and tetanus and has been implicated in cancer, aging, and sudden death. *C. botulinum* produces such deadly poison that one teaspoonful could kill 5 million adults. Another member of the family, *C. perfringens,* causes a particularly nasty case of food poisoning. Face to face with such formidable enemies, you might think that green tea wouldn't have a chance. But when the green tea catechins ECg and EGCg were put to the test against the Clostridium bacteria, they "strongly inhibited" the growth of the bacteria.[3]

Further tests found that catechins could also fight off other bacterial causes of foodborne diseases such as *Plesiomonas shigelloides* (a cause of dysentery), three different *Vibrio* strains (the toxin found in uncooked

1. Toda, 1989.
2. Hara, 1993.
3. Ahn, 1991.

shellfish), *Bacillus cereus*, and *Aeromonas sobria*.[4] And it doesn't take incredible amounts of green tea to do this. In fact, one study found that the concentration of polyphenols in *one cup of tea* was two to three times greater than that needed to kill some bacteria.[5]

Better Than the Pink Stuff

The first mention of tea in Europe occurred in a volume titled *Voyages and Travels*, published in Venice in 1559:

"All over Cathay (China) they made use of another plant . . . called *Chai Catai* (tea of China). . . . They take of that herb, whether dry or fresh, and boil it well in water. One or two cups of this decoction taken on an empty stomach removes fever, headache, stomach ache, pain in the sides or in the joints. . . . It is so highly valued and esteemed that everyone going on a journey takes it with him, and those people would gladly give a sack of rhubarb for one ounce of *Chai Catai*."

—Ramusio,
"Tale of Hajji Mohammed"

But what about the *good* bacteria in the intestine? Does green tea kill them too? Amazingly, the green tea catechins manage to fight deadly bacteria and inhibit the growth of putrefactive bacteria without harming the friendly *bifidus* bacteria.[6]

In fact, the amount of beneficial *acidophillus* bacteria actually *increases* in the presence of green tea. In experiments with 10,000 broiler chickens, half were fed a regular diet and the other half were given the same diet plus 0.07% tea catechins. When ten chickens from each group were sacrificed and their digestive tract contents

4. Ishigami, Food Research Laboratories, Mitsui Norin Co.
5. Toda, 1992.
6. Ishigami., Food Research Laboratories, Mitsui Norin Co.

analyzed, it was found that those who had been fed the tea catechins had *more* beneficial organic acids and acidophillus bacteria.[7]

Similar experiments were conducted on the intestinal bacteria found in chicks. Researchers concluded that green tea catechins not only contributed to the improvement of intestinal flora and environment, but also had a deodorant effect on the chicks' feces.[8] And in tests using pigs, the putrefactive products in their digestive tracts decreased markedly during the time they were fed catechins, but then sharply increased when catechin feeding stopped.[9]

Since green tea inhibits the action of "bad" bacteria and encourages the action of "good" bacteria, it makes sense that it might also help with bowel regularity. To test this theory, thirty-seven people were given tea catechins twice a day (a total of 500 mg daily) for twelve weeks or longer. Just over 50% of the group had regular bowel movements before the experiment began, but over 80% reported regularity at the end of the twelve weeks. Researchers attributed this to the action of the catechins, which helped "to keep the bowel in good condition."[10]

Green Tea, Bacteria, and the Mouth

"Drinking green tea makes the mouth clean."
—Traditional Japanese saying

Green tea's bacteria fighting prowess isn't limited to the digestive system. It also plays an important role in oral hygiene—which translates to fewer cavities,

7. Hara, 1993.
8. Terada, 1993.
9. Hara, 1993.
10. Ishigami, Food Research Laboratories, Mitsui Norin Co.

cleaner, fresher breath, and even protection against root canals! Asians have been drinking tea after meals or after eating sweets for centuries, but we Westerners are only beginning to understand why.

The bacteria primarily responsible for causing dental caries (or "cavities") is *Streptococcus mutans*. These bacteria act on sugars in your mouth to produce a sticky, water-insoluble substance called *glucan* (plaque) that coats the teeth. When microorganisms accumulate on the glucan to feed, they produce acid as a by-product of metabolism, which eats into your tooth enamel and causes dental caries.

In laboratory tests, green tea catechins inhibited the production of plaque by the *S. mutans* bacteria.[11] Other experiments showed that green tea catechins actually destroyed these bacteria, even when the catechins were at concentrations lower than those found in only *one cup of tea.*[12]

Studies showed that Japanese children who drank a cup of green tea immediately after lunch had significantly fewer cavities than those who did not.[13] And bacteria were found to be strongly inhibited after only five to ten minutes of exposure to the tea.[14] In fact, one study concluded that green tea extract was more effective than fluoride compounds in preventing dental caries.[15]

> "Ecstasy is a glass full of tea and a piece of sugar in the mouth."
>
> —Alexander Pushkin

Other kinds of tea have shown similar effects against cavity-producing bacteria. Black, green, oolong, and pu-

11. Hattori, 1990.
12. Sakanaka, 1989.
13. Kada, 1985.
14. Sakanaka, 1989.
15. Hikino, 1985.

erh tea (a Chinese tea known for its medicinal value) all completely inhibit plaque formation by *s. mutans* at concentrations four times less than that found in the average cup of tea. But antibacterial effects were strongest in green tea, followed by pu-erh, black, and oolong.[16]

At least one study found that the theaflavins in black tea were best at inhibiting *S. mutans* activity, but that the EGCg and ECg in green tea were also potent adversaries of plaque formation. And the catechins had the added advantage of being able to prevent bacteria from sticking to the teeth.[17]

Tea is also naturally rich in fluoride, the mineral that many communities add to their water supplies to help prevent cavities. Fluoride interacts with tooth enamel, hardening it and making it 50–70% less susceptible to decay.[18] The amount of fluoride needed to achieve this result (and the amount found in municipal water supplies) is between 0.7 and 1.2 parts per million (PPM). But most green teas sold in the United States contain higher amounts of fluoride than fluoridated water does, usually between 1.32 to 4.18 PPM. Fluoride is toxic in excess, but a person would need to take in between 20 and 80 times the amount found in the average fluoridated water supply for several years before symptoms of toxicity would appear.[19] Thus, it appears that you can drink as much green tea as you want without having to worry about fluoride toxicity.

Whether it's due to fluoride or bacteria-fighting ability, drinking green tea has been found to be a very effective way to protect the teeth from decay. Recently, after many years of research, Dr. Masao Onishi of the Tokyo University of Medicine and Dentistry concluded that drinking just one cup of green tea each day would

16. Ishigami, Food Research Laboratories, Mitsui Norin Co.
17. Hattori, 1990.
18. *The Wellness Encyclopedia*, p. 494.
19. Hamilton, p. 300.

prevent *half* of the reported cases of tooth decay in school-aged children. He said, "Even just rinsing the mouth out with green tea after meals is a highly effective method of preventing tooth decay."

Green tea can also kill other oral bacteria, including some that cause bad breath. It contains the well-known deodorizer chlorophyll, as well as flavonoid, two effective breath fresheners.[20]

And green tea is an effective fighter of certain kinds of bacteria found in infected root canals. Extracts of four kinds of Japanese green tea were tested against twenty-four bacterial strains taken from infected root canals. All four teas showed antibacterial and bactericidal actions against many of the bacterial strains, and completely inhibited eight of those strains *(S. sanguis, P. niger, Ps. anaerobius, Bifid. bifidum, E. lentun, V. parvula, F. nucleatum, and B. endodontalis)*.[21]

Green Tea Against Viruses

Bacteria are not the only microscopic troublemakers. Viruses, tiny microorganisms that "hijack" their host's cells, are the source of some of the most dangerous and communicable diseases in the world, including AIDS. And viruses can attack plants as well as humans and animals. Taking their cue from Japanese tobacco growers who used an extract of green tea to stop the growth of the "tobacco mosaic virus," scientists tested EGCg and ECg against a cell culture that was given a dose of a rotavirus. Both of these catechins inhibited the viral infection of the cells.[22] Since that time, tea leaves have been found to have antiviral activity against the influenza (flu) virus,[23] herpes simplex virus, vaccinia virus,

20. Hainer, 1954.
21. Horiba, 1991.
22. Hatta, 1989.
23. Nakayama, 1990.

Coxsackie virus B6, and polio virus 1,[24] all of which cause serious diseases in humans.

Both green tea catechins and theaflavin from black tea inhibit the influenza virus by preventing it from attaching to cells. (Remember, the virus is most dangerous when it attaches to and "hijacks" your body cells.) The best effects were seen when the tea extracts were added directly to the virus.[25] This means that gargling with green or black tea, and keeping the tea in contact with the virus for as long as possible, is very effective in preventing the flu.[26]

Even more exciting is green tea's possible effect against the AIDS virus. Scientists at the Aichi Cancer Center Research Institute in Nagoya, Japan, found that ECg and EGCg both strongly inhibited the activity of HIV reverse transcriptase, working as well as the well-known drug AZT.[27] Much more research is needed, but it's a promising start.

Green Tea Strengthens the Immune System

In addition to its devastating effect on bacteria and viruses, green tea may help the body fight off invaders by stimulating the immune system to work harder and better. One study revealed that EGCg encourages the production of interleukin-1,[28] which in turn causes an increase in the numbers of T-cells. These T-cells then secrete chemicals that spur giant cell-eating structures called *macrophages* to gobble up foreign invaders.

Another study found that EGCg strengthened the effect of the immune system's B-cells, and caused them to reproduce more rapidly in mice.[29] This is important

24. John, 1979.
25. Mukoyama, 1991.
26. Oguni, *Green Tea and Human Health*.
27. Nakane, 1990.
28. Sakagami, 1992.
29. Hu, 1992.

because just a single B-cell produces thousands and thousands of antibodies, each programmed to attack specific invaders. Anything that increases the strength or number of B-cells can markedly "rev up" the power of the immune system.

Green Tea and Epilepsy

Head injuries are always serious, especially if the brain itself is injured. Trauma to the brain can sometimes bring on epileptic seizures. Searching for a way to help people with brain injuries, scientists induced epilepsy in laboratory rats by giving them injections of iron salts. But when the rats were given EGC before being injected with the iron salts, the green tea catechin *completely prevented the development of epileptic activity*. Treatment with EGC *after* the iron injection also markedly inhibited the development of epileptic symptoms.[30]

> "While there's tea, there's hope."
> —Sir Arthur Pinero

Green Tea Makes Breathing Easier

Certain people carry a form of *Staphylococcus aureus* in their respiratory tracts; this contagious bacteria can be the source of a serious infection. In some cases the drug usually used to knock out this bacteria, Methicillin, doesn't work. If that's the case, the person is said to have Methicillin-resistant *Staphylococcus aureus,* or MRSA. The problem is compounded by the fact that it's difficult to detect, so the disease may go untreated and eventually spread to others. Physicians have been reluctant to use other, stronger antibiotics, because MRSA is already a

30. Mori, 1990.

"strong," resistant strain, and using even more powerful drugs may simply cause the bacteria to become even more resistant. But researchers found that inhaling a solution containing catechins led to a marked decrease in MRSA infection. In a week's time, in fact, most patients were completely free of this bacteria.[31]

Green Tea And Aging

One of the most commonly accepted theories of aging is the *free radical theory* (discussed in Chapter 3). This argues that these unstable molecules careen around the body stealing electrons from other molecules, and generally wreaking havoc. The free radical singlet oxygen turns fats in the body into *peroxide*, triggering cancer, heart disease, diabetes, osteoarthritis, and other diseases associated with advancing age. And the older a person gets, the more the body produces peroxide, and the harder it is to get rid of it.

Many scientists believe that aging can be slowed if free radicals are corralled before they produce too much peroxide. How can we do that? With plenty of antioxidants. Indeed, tests on animals have shown that the higher the concentration of vitamins C and E in their bodies, the longer they live.[32] Drinking green tea may help us fight aging even more effectively than these substances, since the catechins have been shown to be stronger antioxdidants (far stronger, in some cases) than either vitamin E or vitamin C.

One of the common and painful accompaniments to aging, osteoarthritis, may be lessened by drinking green tea, since it's a good source of bioflavonoids. In the bestselling book *The Arthritis Cure*, Dr. Jason Theodosakis states, "Bioflavonoids help to keep the collagen (an important part of the cartilage matrix) strong and

31. Kono, School of Medicine, Fukuoka University, Japan, 1992.
32. Oguni., "Green Tea and Human Health".

resistant to inflammation. They also prevent free radical damage and help to heal damaged tissue following injury."[33] He goes on to name green tea as a food containing good amounts of bioflavonoids. More study must be done, of course, but it seems that green tea may be an excellent "secret weapon" in the war against aging.

Heaven in a Cup

"I am in no way interested in immortality, but only in the taste of tea."

—Lu T'ung

Green Tea as a "Pick-Me-Up"

Ever since eighth-century Buddhist monks discovered that tea helped them remain awake during long meditation sessions, tea has been used to boost lagging energy, refresh the mind, and brighten up the mood. Its stimulating effects are due to caffeine, which is quite possibly the most popular drug in existence. Almost everyone takes in some caffeine on a daily basis via coffee, tea, cola drinks, or chocolate. (The average American tea drinker takes in about 80–100 mg of caffeine per day, while the average coffee drinker takes in twice that.) And the energizing effects are familiar: Heartbeat increases, alertness improves, reaction time gets faster, and the general mood becomes more "upbeat." Some studies have also found that ingestion of caffeine improves reading speed (without increasing errors) and may even heighten intellectual activity.

The downside of caffeine is that too much can cause nervousness, chronic muscle tension, irritability, headaches, depression, and insomnia. Most healthy adults who drink moderate amounts of coffee or tea can handle 200–250 mg of caffeine a day without adverse reactions, but those who aren't used to caffeine or are especially sensitive may get jittery after just one cup of coffee.

> "Tea tempers the spirit and harmonizes the mind; dispels lassitude and relieves fatigue; awakens thought and prevents drowsiness."
>
> —Lu Yu,
> Ch'a Ching

Research into caffeine and its effect on health has been inconclusive. Although there have been some reports of links between caffeine consumption and heart disease, benign breast disease and cancer, studies have not confirmed them. In fact, a recent study conducted in Norway by the National Health Screening Service showed that caffeine was *not* the culprit that caused an increase of heart disease in coffee drinkers. Instead, it was due to the fact that coffee stimulates production of an amino acid called *homocysteine,* which causes plaque to build up on artery walls. For most people, ingesting moderate amounts of caffeine has little or no health risk. Still, many doctors advise people with heart disease, pregnant women, nursing mothers, children, and those who have trouble sleeping to avoid caffeine, or at least limit intake to 200 mg per day. For those who are strictly limiting their intake of caffeine, Opti-Pure offers a completely caffeine-free green tea extract.

Green tea may offer the best of both worlds when it comes to caffeine—just enough to provide a stimulating pick-me-up that banishes unwanted drowsiness, but not enough to trigger nervousness or sleepless nights. The average cup of green tea contains anywhere from 8 to 20 mg of caffeine, while black tea contains at least twice that amount—40 to 60 mg. And a cup of drip coffee has a nerve-jangling 90 to 150 mg, more than half the amount of caffeine that some people should consume in a whole day. Caffeine watchers, take note: It would take at least 4 cups of the strongest green tea to equal the caffeine content of the weakest drip coffee. Still, green tea does have a "brightening" effect.

How Much Caffeine Are You Getting?

If you're concerned about caffeine, use this chart to figure your daily intake. Remember that doctors often recommend no more than 200 mg of caffeine per day.

Beverage	Caffeine, mg
Coffee (5 ounces)	
Drip method	115
Percolated	80
Instant	65
Decaffeinated	3
Green Tea (5 ounces)	
Brewed (3 minutes)	15
Black Tea (5 ounces)	
Brewed (3 minutes)	40
Decaffeinated	5
Iced (12 ounces)	70
Chocolate Beverages	
Cocoa (5 ounces)	4
Chocolate milk (8 ounces)	5
Soft Drinks (12 ounces)	
Coca-Cola	46
Diet Coke	46
Pepsi-Cola	38
Diet Pepsi	40
RC Cola	36
Mountain Dew	54

Source: Food and Drug Administration/National Soft Drink Association.

Other Uses for Green Tea

In today's busy, enterprising world, thousands upon thousands of products sit on shelves in grocery stores, drugstores, pharmacies, and department stores just waiting to be purchased. Sometimes they wait a long time, which is why manufacturers are quite concerned about keeping perishable items such as food and cosmetics fresh.

Antioxidants have been used for years to preserve the freshness of foods and cosmetics, especially those containing fats or oils, which can quickly become rancid. And guess what's the latest, greatest new thing for extending the shelf-life of perishable items? Our old friend, green tea. And why not? Green tea gives potent antioxidant protection, it fights bacteria, its extract is very stable in both liquid and powder form, and it has absolutely no chemical side effects or other threats to good health. Manufacturers are just beginning to catch the green tea wave, but most likely you'll start to see it popping up just about everywhere very soon, playing one of the following roles:

- *Food Preservative.* To preserve the freshness of fats and oils, food manufacturers have long relied on the use of vitamins C and E. But even though these vitamins are very effective at preventing the spoilage of fats and oils, studies show that green tea extract has much more potent anti-rancidity activity than either of them. In fact, green tea extract is ten times more effective than vitamin E and 2.5 times more potent than a fat-soluble form of vitamin C at preventing oils and fats from "turning bad." Green tea extract even works in oil exposed to sunlight, oil solubilized in water, and when vitamin E and the preservative BHA (commonly used in baked goods to prevent rancidity) are completely ineffective.[34]

In one study, the catechins were tested individually in vegetable oils. Four of them—EC, EGC, ECg, and EGCg—inhibited spoilage due to oxidation. EGCg was

34. Food Research Laboratories: Tea and Health.

found to be 200 times more potent an antioxidant than vitamin E, the "gold standard" of oil preservatives.[35] Some seafood dealers are now considering dipping their fish and other fresh products in a mixture of green tea extract and water to keep them fresher for longer periods of time. Today, green tea extract is widely used in the food industry in Japan as a preservative in products containing fats and oils such as fish, baked goods, margarine, and bottled oils.

• *Food Additive.* Would you believe a green tea chocolate bar? Distributed by Cloud Nine, Inc. of Hoboken, New Jersey, it contains organic dairy-free chocolate, puffed basmati rice, and green tea extract. There is also a hard candy made from green tea (by Garden of Songs, c/o Vision 21 Marketing in Morristown, New Jersey) and a frozen fruit bar made from green tea and fruit juice (by Tazo of Portland, Oregon). And don't be surprised to find green tea popping up in many other foods in the very near future. Because of its anticancer, antibacterial, antiviral, and heart protective effects, green tea extract may soon be added to various processed foods such as pasta, bread, cereal, muffins, or other items to enhance health. The liquid or powder forms of the extract can be easily added to just about any food without compromising taste or quality.

• *Cosmetic Ingredient.* Many kinds of makeup, lotions, creams, and other beauty preparations contain oil, so antioxidants must be added to preserve their freshness. Oxidation of cosmetics can make them not only ineffective and smelly, but can cause the formation of potentially dangerous substances. Many cosmetic manufacturers use chemical preservatives such as methylparaben or propylparaben to extend the shelf life of their products. But manufacturers of "natural" cosmetics usually stick with natural preservatives like the antioxidant vitamins A, C, and E, even though they're not as powerful as the chemicals. Green tea extract, though, has been

35. Uchida, 1990.

proven to be an even stronger antioxidant than these powerful vitamins in some cases, and is, of course, totally natural. It's also an excellent antibacterial agent with both anti-inflammatory and anti-irritancy effects.

Green tea also may lend "anti-aging" properties to cosmetics thanks to its ability to scavenge free radicals. Fighting free radicals from within the body seems to be an effective way to slow down the aging process, but there is still some question as to whether fighting them from without by applying antioxidants to the skin will do the same thing. But whether or not it can truly fight aging, green tea extract is fast becoming the new "designer" cosmetic ingredient found in all kinds of products from facial scrubs to eye creams.

Replacing vitamin E, which was long the most popular antioxidant in the beauty field, green tea is the "new kid on the block" that everyone hopes will be a powerful tool in the never-ending war against aging and UV damage. Some of the new products that contain green tea extract include:

Facial Cleansers

- *Sugar Cane and Meadowsweet Alpha-Hydroxy Facial Scrub* (by Freeman)
- *Green Tea & Chamomile Soap* (by Primal Elements)
- *Green Tea Facial Cleansing Lotion* (by Aubrey Organics)

Moisturizers and Creams

- *Beta-Ginseng Age-Protective Anti-Oxidant Eye Gel* (by Earth Science)
- *Tea Time Anti-Aging Moisturizing Creme* (by Jason Natural Cosmetics)
- *Urban Defense Cream* (by D'Arcy)
- *Green Tea Nourishing Eye Gel* (by Beauty Without Cruelty)
- *Green Tea & Ginkgo Daily Moisturizer SPF 15* (by Aubrey Organics)

- *Phytosome Nutrient Infusion* (by Primal Elements)
- *Eye Doctor Eye Cream* (by Origins)
- *Green Tea Hand & Body Lotion with Evening Primrose* (by Aubrey Organics)

Sunblock

- *Green Tea Sunblock for Children (SPF 25)* (by Aubrey Organics)

Facial Toners and Masks

- *Green Tea & Green Clay Rejuvenating Facial Mask* (by Aubrey Organics)
- *Sugar Cane and Guava Alpha-Hydroxy Peel-Off Masque* (by Freeman)
- *Alpha Natural Skin Renewal Facial Mask* (by Naturistics)
- *Green Tea & Ginkgo Facial Toner* (by Aubrey Organics)

Hair Care Products

- *Green Tea Hair Treatment Shampoo* (by Aubrey Organics)
- *Green Tea Herbal Cream Rinse* (by Aubrey Organics)

Fragrance

- *Eau Parfumee Extreme*—a unisex green tea fragrance (by Bulgari, the jewelers).

Toothpaste/Mouthwash

Given green tea's ability to prevent dental caries by fighting *Streptococcus mutans* and other bacteria in the mouth, it's only natural that it be used in oral hygiene products. Green tea prevents plaque-causing bacteria from attaching to dental surfaces, and it follows that toothpaste and mouthwash containing green tea would have the same effect. It also inhibits the growth of several other kinds of odor-producing bacteria in the mouth, and its chlorophyll is a natural breath freshener. Chemco Industries produces both a mouthwash and a chewable breath freshener that contain the green tea extract Polyphenon 60™.

Deodorant

A couple of new deodorants containing green tea are now available. *Wild Yam 5% Clear and Natural Deodorant* (by Woman Wise™) contains green tea extract, vitamin E, and extracts of grape seed, litchen, and horsetail. Touted as an antioxidant formula that neutralizes odor and protects against perspiration, this formula shuns the ingredients typically found in deodorants—aluminum chlorhydrate, alcohol, and chemical bactericides—while promising long-lasting natural protection.

• *Green Tea, Vitamin E & Calendula Natural Deodorant* (Aubrey Organics) is formulated for children or adults with sensitive skin. Antioxidant action is provided by the green tea and vitamin E. Both the tea and the calendula blossom oil found in the deodorant have antibacterial and antifungal properties that help control perspiration odor. As with all other Aubrey Green Tea products, the tea used is matcha, a high grade of tea that may contain greater amounts of catechins.

Weight Loss Aid

Studies show that taking green tea twice a day can help reduce the formation of excess fat cells and curb appetite. Dr. Tsang-do Houng, a researcher at the University of Beijing and graduate of Harvard Medical School, says "A cup twenty minutes before a meal makes you feel filled up and kills hunger pangs."

When rats were fed a normal diet plus green tea extract, the accumulation of body fat was suppressed and they got thinner. But when the extract was used over a long period of time, the fat reduction leveled off, so that body fat stores did not become abnormally low.[36]

36. Mitsui Norin Co., Ltd., "Polyphenon 60."

Diet teas are all the rage with dieters because they fill the stomach while soothing and relaxing. Since tea must be sipped slowly, the dieter learns to slow down and take small mouthfuls, techniques that help one lose weight. At least one "dieter's tea" currently on the market (Hobe Laboratories' *Thermo Slim Tea*) is based on green tea. It also contains "thermogenic herbs" believed to increase the amount of heat generated by the body, thus increasing calorie expenditure.

A Means of Maintaining the Body's Fluid Balance

Water is an integral part of the human body, so essential that we can survive only a few days without it. A full 60% of the body is made up of water, and it constitutes a large part of every single cell. Water is the transport vehicle for both nutrients and waste products, providing the cells with nourishment as well as a "sanitation system." Because water resists compression, its presence in and around the cells, tissues, and organs helps ensure that they don't press too hard against each other or "wear away" because of friction. And water responds slowly to changes in temperature, so it helps keep internal heat at a constant level.

Obviously, maintaining the body's water balance by drinking plenty of fluid is vital for good health. Many of the world's people rely heavily on tea for the bulk of their fluid intake—an excellent choice since it brings with it so many health-giving substances. Vitamins, minerals, catechins, flavonoids, fluoride, and caffeine are just some of the valuable "extras" that tea drinkers ingest along with their favorite beverage. And since these health-boosting ingredients exist in a water base, the body can absorb them more completely.

In a Nutshell: Green Tea's Health Benefits

Green tea has been highly regarded for thousands of years as a healing medicinal beverage. And in recent years, scientists have confirmed the validity of its ancient reputation, discovering that green tea can fight disease and even lengthen life by:

- Preventing normal cells from turning cancerous.
- Suppressing the formation and growth of tumors.
- Guarding against free radical damage that can bring about cancer, heart disease, diabetes, radiation damage, and aging.
- Enhancing immune system function.
- Controlling cholesterol levels.
- Lowering the risk of stroke by making blood platelets less "sticky."
- Controlling blood pressure levels.
- Keeping blood sugar at moderate levels.
- Fighting deadly food-borne bacteria.
- Promoting "friendly" bacteria in the intestines and encouraging bowel regularity.
- Fighting viruses, including those that cause herpes simplex, polio, and even HIV.
- Lowering the risk of post-traumatic epileptic seizures in laboratory animals.
- Assisting in weight loss by blocking the breakdown of starch.
- Providing a mild stimulating effect without causing sleepless nights or nervousness.
- Fighting bacteria in the mouth that cause cavities and bad breath.
- Slowing the aging process.
- Maintaining the body's fluid balance.
- Reducing stress.
- Acting as a safe and effective natural preservative in food and cosmetics.

No other substance on the face of the earth, including the most potent drug, can claim such wide-ranging and powerful health benefits, *and all without a single side effect*. Yes, green tea can truly perform "miracles" for just pennies a cup.

CHAPTER 6

Does Black Tea Have Any Health Benefits?

This admirable drink reconciles men to sobriety.
—John Ovington, regarding tea
Eighteenth-century English parson

Clearly, green tea is a powerful weapon against several deleterious diseases and conditions. But how about black tea? Does it also promote good health?

Black tea has long been used as a medicine, a pleasing beverage, and a psychologically soothing tonic. Not surprisingly, scientists have discovered that black tea *does* have several health benefits, although they are not nearly as wide-ranging and powerful as those of green tea. That's because most of green tea's health-promoting characteristics come from catechins, which are mostly oxidized into theaflavins and thearubigens during the manufacture of black tea. These new compounds do have some of their own health benefits, but they can't compare with the wide-ranging effects of green tea's catechins, especially the powerful EGCg.

Still, the theaflavins and thearubigens are strong antioxidants, and worthy of serious attention. Let's take a look at several of black tea's health benefits.

EGCg Content

While a cup of black tea contains about 5–10 mg of the powerful catechin EGCg, a cup of green tea contains more than *eight times that amount,* or 40–90 mg.

Tea and Cancer

Scientists at Rutgers University have recently shown that both green and black teas can protect against the development of skin cancer in mice. The animals' skins were treated with a carcinogen, then they were exposed to UVB (ultaviolet-B) light. Those who were also given either green or black tea developed 65–93% fewer carcinomas and 60–90% fewer skin tumors than those who were not given tea.[1]

In a test of various kinds of tea extracts, both black and green tea inhibited the promotion of laboratory-induced tumors in mice by about 70%.[2] Both of these teas have also been found to block the formation of nitrosamines (powerful carcinogens that are assembled within the body) as well as nitrosamine-induced tumors of the stomach and intestines.[3] And black tea was as effective as green tea in inhibiting the formation of lung and esophageal tumors in laboratory animals injected with a potent carcinogen found in cigarette smoke.[4]

Black tea showed its medicinal muscle in laboratory studies, but would it protect humans as well? The answer is yes, according to a study that compared the cancer rates of black tea drinkers with non–tea drinkers in a group of 35,369 postmenopausal women in Iowa. (Those who drank only herbal tea were not considered

1. Wang, 1994.
2. Nakamura, 1991.
3. Yang, 1993.
4. Ibid.

tea drinkers in this study.) Among the women who drank two or more cups of tea per day, there was a 10% reduction in all types of cancer; 32% fewer cancers of the upper digestive tract, colon, and rectum; and a 60% reduction in urinary tract cancer. Even better, those who drank four cups of tea or more daily showed a 60% reduction in all of these cancers.[5]

Tea, Heart Disease, and Stroke

A Dutch study completed in 1990 followed 805 men, aged sixty-five to eighty-four, for five years, studying their intake of the antioxidant-rich flavonoids (found in abundance in tea, vegetables, fruits, and wine) and the effect on their death rate from coronary heart disease. Most of the flavonoids in the men's diets (61%) came from black tea, while 13% came from onions and 10% from apples. After five years, the study found that there was a strong link between a high flavonoid intake and a lower risk of death due to heart disease. This study certainly suggests that black tea has a protective effect on the heart.[6]

A similar study, again from the Netherlands, this time lasting for fifteen years, found that those with a high intake of flavonoids had *a 73% lower risk of stroke.* When researchers adjusted the results to allow them to look at the effects of tea alone, they found that those who drank more than 4.7 cups per day had a 69% reduced risk of stroke, compared to those who drank less than 2.6 cups. The researchers concluded that the habitual intake of flavonoids and their major source (tea) could protect against strokes.[7]

5. Zheng, 1996.
6. Hertog, 1993.
7. Keli, 1996.

Tea and the Liver

It appears that both black and green tea can help the body purify itself. Both teas were found to be equally powerful in increasing the metabolic processes by which rat livers detoxify carcinogens and other toxins. This makes the liver better able to inactivate these poisons and excrete them, theoretically reducing the risk of cancer and other ailments.[8]

Tea, the Antioxidant

Even though black tea lacks the powerful antioxidant action of the catechins, its theaflavins and thearubigens exert their own mighty antioxidant punch. Scientists at Rutgers University found that gallic acid, a substance found in black tea, could strongly inhibit the oxidation of lard.[9] A Japanese study done in 1994 found that theaflavins helped protect the membranes of rabbit blood cells from oxidation damage, while warding off much of the damaging effects of hydrogen peroxide on DNA.[10] And yet another Japanese study found that theaflavins and thearubigens in black tea inhibited the oxidation of fatty substances in rat livers just as well as EGCg, and even better than vitamin E or vitamin C.[11]

This ability to block the oxidation of fats is probably the reason that black tea lowered the risk of strokes and death from heart disease in the Dutch studies. The flavonoids also blocked the oxidation of the LDL, which has long been considered to be one of the early events in coronary artery disease.[12]

8. Sohn, 1994.
9. Ho, 1992.
10. Shiraki, 1994.
11. Yoshino, 1994.
12. Keli, 1996.

Tea and Kidney Stones

Although patients with kidney stones are almost always advised to increase their intake of fluids, only recently have researchers tried to figure out just which drinks were most likely to prevent the stones—or cause them to form in the first place. At the Johns Hopkins University School of Hygiene and Public Health, scientists studied the relationship between twenty-one different beverages and kidney stone formation in 45,289 men. (Ranging in age from forty to seventy-five, none of them had a history of kidney stones.) The results were intriguing, showing that each 8-ounce serving of black tea consumed daily led to a 14% decrease in the risk of stone formation.[13]

Tea and Skin Inflammation

Black tea is high in astringent tannins, which can help relieve skin inflammation. Cool, wet tea bags have long been applied to soothe burns, and a quart of strong black tea added to a lukewarm bath can be an effective remedy for sunburn.

Tea and Diarrhea

Black tea's theaflavins and thearubigens appear to have a calming, soothing effect on the stomach and intestines that may make the brew an effective remedy for diarrhea. In fact, doctors and mothers have known for years that kids with diarrhea should be put on the BRAT diet (bananas, rice, applesauce, and tea).

Tea and Tooth Decay

All teas are good sources of fluoride, the mineral that hardens tooth enamel. And even though black tea

13. Curhan, 1996.

contains only about half the amount of fluoride found in green tea, just one cup per day may confer powerful protection against cavities. Like green tea, black tea can interfere with the formation of plaque and fight oral bacteria, and is most effective when sipped at the end of a meal.

Tea Is Good for You

In short, it appears that *any* brew made from the *Camellia sinensis* bush is good for you. Although black tea doesn't appear to wield quite the health-promoting punch that green tea does, it certainly qualifies as a "steaming cup of medicine" all on its own.

The First Tea Bag

The first tea bag was invented in 1904 by New Yorker Thomas Sullivan, a resourceful tea and coffee merchant. Ordinarily he sent small tins of loose tea to his customers as samples, but after a while this began to get expensive. Sullivan decided to put the tea into little handmade silk bags instead. Soon the customers discovered that they could leave the tea leaves in the bags, pour boiling water over them, and make tea with less muss and fuss. No messy straining! The orders for Sullivan's little bags of tea began to pour in. Today about 95% of America's hot tea comes from tea bags, and many people have never had their tea any other way.

CHAPTER 7

The Marriage of Green Tea and Other Ingredients

If a man has no tea in him, he is incapable of understanding truth and beauty.

—Ancient Japanese saying

All by itself, green tea offers a mind-boggling range of health benefits. It's incredible to think that this single substance can, among other things, fight both cancer and heart disease, lower high blood sugar, inhibit bacteria and viruses, slow the aging process, and ward off viruses and bacteria. All this, and in such a delicious and satisfying form! What more could anyone possibly want?

Nothing—unless maybe someone could find a way to make tea's health-promoting effects even stronger.

Heeding the call, many manufacturers are now adding herbs, vitamins, and extracts that are themselves powerful health aids to their green tea. Some of these additives reinforce green tea's existing medicinal effects, others add new ones. Here are some of the many ingredients that you might find added to your green tea, and what they may do for your health:

Aloe Vera *(Aloe vera)*

The gel taken from the aloe vera leaf is well known for its soothing effect on burned skin. Recently, however, it was also found to be a potent immune booster. In a study performed at Texas A&M University, mice that were implanted with cancerous tumors were 40% less likely to die if they had previously been given oral doses of aloe vera.[1] Aloe taken internally can also act as a mild laxative.

Angelica *(Angelica archangelica)*

Native to Syria, the bark, root, and berries of this herb have expectorant properties that make them good remedies for colds and coughs. Angelica is also used to treat diseases of the urinary system, reduce fevers, promote circulation, relieve cramps, and ease rheumatism.

Astragalus *(Astragalus membranaceus)*

One of the most famous herbs used in Chinese medicine, astragalus is used to increase resistance to disease, while boosting the body's vital energy. Used traditionally in exhausting or wasting diseases as a restorative tonic, it has impressed modern researchers with its ability to strengthen immune function, promote the healing of ulcers, and decrease susceptibility to colds. Its diuretic effect (flushing excess fluids from the body) produces a therapeutic sweating of toxins.

Bilberry *(Vaccinium myrtillus)*

Grown in Europe and Asia and similar to our blueberry, the bilberry contains compounds called *anthocyanides* that may help preserve vision. During World War

1. Mindell, p. 20.

II, Royal Air Force pilots who ate sandwiches spread with bilberry jam just before their night flights claimed that their night vision improved. And studies done in France in 1964 found that bilberry improved the eye's ability to adapt from bright light to darkness. Since then, anthocyanides have been proven to speed up the production of *retinol purple,* a necessary ingredient for good night vision.

Bilberry's anthocyanides are also useful for strengthening the capillary and blood vessel walls, protecting against vascular disease, hemorrhaging, and aneurysm.

Bioflavonoids

The bioflavonoids (sometimes referred to as simply "flavonoids") are a group of some 500 compounds found in the white part of citrus peel, in red and yellow onions, apricots, buckwheat and rose hip tea. Once thought to be nothing more than just a kind of natural "food dye," the bioflavonoids work synergistically with vitamin C to strengthen the walls of the capillaries and small blood vessels, inhibit the action of certain carcinogens and tumor promoters, slow the onset of atherosclerosis by preventing the oxidation of LDL, and fight viruses.

Cardamom *(Elettaria cardamomum)*

One of the first spices exported from East India, cardamom has an exotic gingery-peppery aroma and is used to flavor teas, coffee, and Scandinavian coffee cakes. Cardamom seeds are rich in volatile oils that help stimulate the digestive process and ease flatulence, while soothing stomach and intestinal walls.

Cascara Sagrada *(Rhamnus purshianus)*

Also known as California buckthorn, the bark of this shrub is a digestive system stimulant and one of nature's gentlest, safest laxatives. Cascara sagrada may also help to treat liver problems, colitis, and hemorrhoids.

Cat's Claw Bark Extract *(Uncaria tomentosa)*

The *Uncaria tomentosa* plant is a woody vine native to the Peruvian rainforest that takes its name (cat's claw, or *una de gato*) from the two curved thorns situated at the base of each of its leaves. For generations, the Ashanica Indians made a tea from the bark and root of the cat's claw vine to treat colds, tumors, cold sores, and other conditions. Modern-day scientists have found that it has antioxidant, antiviral, and antitumor properties.

Studies conducted by scientists the world over have found that cat's claw may help treat allergies, diabetes, PMS, arthritis, bursitis, and organic depression. Its immune-strengthening abilities make it an effective weapon against genital herpes, herpes zoster, systemic candidiasis, lupus, chronic fatigue syndrome, and the HIV virus. And its strong antioxidant properties help in warding off cancer, heart problems, aging, and other diseases.

Chamomile *(Matricaria chamomilla)*

One of the oldest garden herbs, a tonic made from chamomile flowers has long been used to relieve tension and stress, while easing sleeplessness. It also encourages the sweating out of toxic substances and may help soothe upset stomachs. Chamomile has been helpful in treating back pain, menstrual cramps, and urinary problems. It may also help to break a high fever.

Chicory *(Cichorium intybus)*

A tonic made from the root of this versatile plant helps to increase the flow of bile, thereby aiding digestion. It may also discourage the formation of gallstones and, thanks to its ability to eliminate uric acid from the body, has been used to treat both rheumatism and gout. Modern research has shown that chicory has anti-inflammatory properties and may be of use in treating irregular and/or rapid heartbeat. Chicory also lowers blood sugar. The roasted roots of the chicory plant are sometimes used as a substitute for coffee, while boiled roots are considered a delicacy in the Middle East.

The Everything Drink

"If you are cold, tea will warm you;
if you are too heated, it will cool you;
if you are depressed, it will cheer you;
if you are exhausted, it will calm you."
—William Gladstone,
British Prime Minister

Chromium Picolinate

A form of the trace mineral chromium, this substance is believed to encourage the building of muscle mass. (Be advised, though, that it only does so in conjunction with exercise!) Chromium also works with insulin to help your body use blood glucose and break down fat, and may be of use in weight loss. Some studies have also suggested that chromium picolinate can help prevent diabetes and heart disease.

Cinnamon *(Cinnamomum zeylanicum)*

Besides the delicious sweet and pungent flavor that cinnamon adds to any food or drink, current Japanese research suggests that it can lower high blood pressure. It has been successfully used to treat colds, ease flatulence, control diarrhea, and soothe menstrual cramps. The oil of cinnamon bark also has antibacterial action, fighting *Staphylococcus aureus, E. coli,* and thrush.

Citrus Terpenes *(Limonene)*

Terpenes are a group of plant compounds with antioxidant properties that help deactivate carcinogens, prevent or slow the growth of certain types of cancer, and control the production of cholesterol. Limonene, a member of the terpene group found in the oil of citrus fruit peels, has been shown to shrink mammary tumors in rats, while preventing the growth of new ones.

Devil's Claw *(Harpagophytum procumbens)*

Devil's claw contains a substance that reduces inflammation in the joints, so it's not surprising that an infusion made from this plant's root is an old folk remedy for arthritis, rheumatism, and gout. It is also used to eliminate uric acid from the body, to purify the blood, and treat liver and gallbladder problems.

Dong Quai Root *(Angelica sinensis)*

Also called "women's ginseng," dong quai is widely used in China to regulate estrogen levels. Its hormone-like compounds relieve menstrual disorders and ease the symptoms of menopause. Dong quai is also highly regarded as an anti-aging herb that can lower both the pulse rate and blood pressure. A rich source of vitamin E as well as iron, this herb can help prevent anemia, act as an antioxidant, and help to regulate blood sugar. Because it acts as a mild sedative and "smoothes out" the emotions, it may also be prescribed for stress and sleeping problems.

Echinacea *(Echinacea angustifolia or Echinacea purpurea)*

Native Americans used the root of this plant, which is also known as the purple coneflower, to treat sore throats, toothaches, and snakebites. They believed that it had more healing uses than any other plant. Over the past fifty years, research has shown that echinacea is a potent immune system booster. It contains a natural antibiotic and increases the production of infection-fighting T-cells, making it effective in the treatment of colds, flu, tonsillitis, bronchitis, and tuberculosis. Echinacea also fights viral infections, inhibits the growth of certain types of tumors, and lessens inflammation.

Elderberry *(Sambucus nigra)*

A good source of both vitamin C and bioflavonoids, elderberries can be useful in the treatment of colds, flu, hayfever, and sinusitis. Especially when taken in a hot infusion (such as tea), elderberry can induce the sweating of poisons while reducing mucous production in the upper respiratory tract. It also has a mild laxative effect.

Eucommia Bark *(Eucommia ulmoidis)*

Herbalists use a tonic made from eucommia bark to energize the kidneys and liver, strengthen the muscles and bones, and increase overall vitality. It is used by the Chinese to lower the blood pressure, and to treat impotence or other sexual dysfunction. Eucommia bark also helps to calm the emotions and is sometimes used to prevent miscarriage.

Feverfew *(Tanacetum parthenium)*

In 1988, the prestigious medical journal *Lancet* published a study verifying the ability of this herb to reduce both the occurrence and severity of migraine headaches. Headache sufferers may find relief after chewing just a few feverfew leaves. Feverfew may also help to lower high blood pressure, alleviate indigestion and gas, lessen anxiety, and relieve menstrual cramps.

Danger: Dirth of Tea

"We had a kettle, we let it leak;
  Our not replacing it made it worse,
We haven't had any tea for a
week . . .
  The bottom is out of the Universe!"
        —Rudyard Kipling,
        Natural Theology

Ginger Root *(Zingiber officinale)*

Ginger is an excellent digestive aid, promoting the secretion of gastric juices, enhancing the absorption of food, and easing indigestion, colic, and flatulence. It also helps alleviate nausea, including the morning sickness of early pregnancy and motion sickness.

Ginger has also shown potent cancer-fighting potential in laboratory tests, and effectively inhibits platelet aggregation. It has anti-inflammatory, antibacterial, antiviral, and antifungal properties that help stimulate immunity. An expectorant, ginger also helps to ease cold symptoms.

Ginkgo Biloba *(Ginkgo biloba)*

Ginkgo biloba, an extract derived from the leaves of the ginkgo tree, is widely used in Europe to treat a variety of conditions, including memory loss. By inhibiting the clumping of platelets that cause plaque to accumulate on artery walls, ginkgo biloba increases the flow of blood to the brain. This helps to improve the memory and increase alertness.[2] Ginkgo may also increase the rate at which information is retrieved from the brain. After taking the extract, reaction time in healthy young subjects became faster,[3] and in elderly subjects mental performance and concentration improved to nearly normal levels.[4]

Ginkgo biloba is rich in flavonoids, making it a potent antioxidant that can help ward off cancer, heart disease, and other conditions caused by free radical damage. It may also help relieve some of the symptoms of asthma, and has been used with some success in treating ringing in the ears (tinnitus), headaches, vertigo, depression, and hemorrhoids.

Ginseng *(Panax Ginseng)*

Panax means "panacea," or a remedy for all ills, and *ginseng* means "man root" because its shape resembles a person. Panax ginseng may not be a cure for every ailment that strikes man, but in traditional Chinese medicine it is prescribed to boost the immune system, strengthen the body's resistance to stress-related illnesses, increase vitality, and treat chronic conditions.

Ginseng is used primarily for exhaustion, depression, or debility, especially in the elderly, the stressed, and those weakened by disease. Some claim that besides increasing vitality, ginseng is also an aphrodisiac. Ginseng is often combined with other herbs, such as Chinese dates or licorice, to tone down its powerful effects, as it can sometimes cause anxiety. *(Note:* Do not take in cases of bronchitis or severe inflammatory disease, for it may make these conditions worse. Also, ginseng causes

2. Murray, *Encyclopedia of Natural Medicine*, pp. 133–134.
3. Hindmarch, 1984.
4. Gebner, 1985.

headaches in certain individuals.) Ginseng is also known as Chinese, Japanese, or Korean ginseng.

Goldenseal Root *(Hydratis canadensis)*

A famous North American Indian medicine, this herb is used to treat inflammation of the mucous membranes, including peptic ulcers. It is also a soothing ingredient found in many lotions. Modern research has confirmed that goldenseal also has antibacterial and antiviral action. External washes containing goldenseal can help heal skin infections, and a gargle made from this herb is good for infected gums and sore throats.

Green Tea Extract

As you know by now, green tea offers a whole host of health benefits. But many studies have found that it takes anywhere from 5 to 20 cups of green tea per day before positive effects on the health begin to show up. However, adding green tea extract can make a single cup of green tea as catechin-rich as 20 cups of regular green tea! Since there is no toxicity associated with the intake of green tea or its extract, it's safe to drink as much as you want. *(See* the Appendix for information on how to find a good extract.)

Gymnema Sylvestre

Used medicinally for centuries in India as a treatment for diabetes, Gymnema Sylvestre is an herb that suppresses the taste of sugar when taken before a meal. People tend to eat less when they can't taste sugar, and several studies have confirmed that this herb can significantly reduce appetite. Not only does Gymnema Sylvestre block the taste of sugar, it also blocks its absorption in the intestines, making it a boon to weight watchers and sugarholics everywhere.

Kava Kava *(Piper methysticum)*

Studies have shown that this shrub, a native of the South Pacific, contains substances that promote relaxation of the muscles and nervous system, producing a dreamy state. For centuries, the natives have boiled the kava kava root to make an alcoholic beverage used in religious and cultural ceremonies. Today in Europe, it is used as the basis of a sedative. Herbalists use kava kava to treat anxiety, nervousness, and sleeplessness.

Kombucha *(Fungus japonicus)*

Kombucha, the "Manchurian tea mushroom," is really not a mushroom at all, but a colony of yeast and bacteria that grows on sweetened tea, forming a jelly-like skin. Many health benefits have been attributed to kombucha, a popular folk remedy for thousands of years, but they have not yet been scientifically proven. Further study will reveal whether kombucha cures cancer, baldness, gout, rheumatism, constipation, irritability, atherosclerosis, and high blood pressure and restores diminished sex drive, as has been claimed.

Kombucha does provide nutrition in the form of amino acids and B vitamins, and can inhibit the growth of certain bacteria. Some people taking kombucha prophylactically have reported catching fewer colds than usual, and kombucha tea may aid digestion. More research is needed before any real claims can be made.

Lemongrass Oil *(Citronella)*

A flavoring used in Asian cooking, lemongrass oil may help lower cholesterol and prevent heart disease.

In one study coming from the University of Wisconsin, men who had high cholesterol took 140 mg of lemongrass oil for three months. Cholesterol levels dropped by 10% in 30% of the subjects. Researchers concluded that lemongrass oil lowered cholesterol by interfering with the production of cholesterol from fats.[5]

Better Than a Good Friend

"What part of confidante has that poor teapot played ever since the kindly plant was introduced among us. . . . What sickbeds it has smoked by! What fevered lips have received refreshment from it!"

—William Makepeace Thackeray,
Pendennis, 1848

Licorice *(Glycyrrhiza glabra)*

Licorice has been used for centuries to ease sore throats and soothe stomach ulcers; in fact, a packet of licorice sticks was found in King Tut's tomb! Tea made from this sweet, slightly musky-tasting root was used by Native Americans as both a laxative and a cough medicine because of its ability to both soothe and coat. (Although licorice candy is a well-known sweet, it actually contains no licorice at all. Instead, the candy is flavored with anise oil, which has a similar taste.) Almost 90% of the licorice imported by the United States is used for one purpose—to add flavor to cigarette tobacco!

One of the main constituents of licorice is *glycyrrhizin*, which is fifty times sweeter than sugar, making licorice root an excellent sweetener that can mask the bitter taste of other herbs in tea. Herbalists recommend licorice as an expectorant, an anti-inflammatory agent, and a treatment for adrenal problems, heartburn, ulcers, and

5. Mindell, pp. 99–100.

colic. Licorice is also used to regulate estrogen levels, but too much of it can cause water retention.

Ling Chih Mushroom *(Ganoderma Lucidum)*

Also known as the "plant of immortality," this Chinese mushroom has been used in the folk medicine of Japan and China for 4,000 years to treat kidney disease, high blood pressure, bronchitis, asthma, and ulcers.

Laboratory studies have shown that the Ling Chih mushroom can stimulate the immune system, slow or halt tumor growth, lower blood pressure, lessen the severity of bronchitis and asthma attacks, inhibit allergic reactions, ease pain, and fight viruses and bacteria.

Lobelia *(Lobelia inflata)*

Lobelia, also known as Indian tobacco, is used to treat muscle spasms and sprains by relaxing surrounding tissues. North American Indians used to smoke lobelia instead of tobacco, and it is sometimes used today to ease tobacco withdrawal symptoms. It is also an effective expectorant, useful in the treatment of asthma and bronchitis.

Lycii Fruit *(Litchi chinensis)*

Also called the lycii nut, this member of the soap-berry family has a tough, scaly skin surrounding soft edible flesh that holds a small hard seed. In Chinese medicine, lyciis (either fresh or dried) are used to treat hiccuping, asthma, digestive problems, and hernial pain. A brew made from lycii seeds and fresh ginger or dried orange peel is used to relieve stomach aches. A soup made from lycii seeds and caraway seeds is believed to relieve hernial pain, swelling of the testes, and elephantiasis.

Ma Huang *(Ephedra sinica)*

This herb is a powerful diaphoretic (sweat-inducer) meant to help the body release toxins. It is also used to relieve congested breathing passages. Acting as a stimulant, Ma Huang speeds up the metabolism and raises the blood pressure, and has recently become a popular addition to many diet aids and "pep" pills. Be aware that the use of this herb can result in headaches, dizziness, or rapid heartbeat in sensitive individuals.

Maitake Mushroom *(Grifola frondosa)*

"Maitake" means "dancing mushroom" in Japanese, and some say it got this name because in ancient times the mushroom could be exchanged for its weight in silver, making those who found it dance with happiness. For hundreds of years, this mushroom has been prized by Japanese herbologists for its ability to beef up the immune system and strengthen overall health.

A number of studies have found maitake mushrooms to be potent cancer fighters, showing an antitumor effect,[6] stimulating the T-cells (the body's natural killer cells), and generally enhancing the immune system. Laboratory studies with animals have demonstrated maitake's other health benefits: it reduces blood pressure (without affecting HDL levels), protects kidney cells from damage, and lowers blood glucose levels in diabetic rats.[7]

Maitake also helps inhibit weight gain. Rats that would normally be expected to gain 130–240 g in one month of continuous feeding gained only 20–30 g when their feed included 20% dried maitake powder.[8] In human trials done at the Koseikai Clinic in Tokyo, Japan, thirty patients were given twenty 500 mg tablets

6. Adachi, 1987.
7. Nariba, 1994.
8. Ohtsuru, 1992.

of powdered maitake each day with no change in their diets. After two months, all of the patients had lost weight, with an average loss of 11–13 pounds.[9]

When used regularly (3–5 times a week) in tea, in supplement form, or in cooking, maitake may help prevent cancer, enhance the immune system, encourage weight loss, and help to lower both high blood sugar and elevated blood pressure.

Milk Thistle (Silybum marianum)

The seeds of the milk thistle plant have long been used to treat digestive disorders and liver conditions. Milk thistle contains a compound called silymarin, which stimulates the secretion of bile from the liver and gallbladder, aiding digestion. The liver, the body's major detoxifying organ, is exposed to many poisons: milk thistle contains chemical components that help protect liver cells from the dangerous effects of these toxins. In Europe, milk thistle has been used successfully to treat a variety of liver disorders, including hepatitis and cirrhosis.

Pai Shu Root (Atractylodes macrocephala)

Pai shu is given as a diuretic tonic to eliminate excess water, sodium, and other electrolytes. Gentler on the kidneys than other diuretics, pai shu is also used for diarrhea, indigestion, bloating, vomiting, and abdominal distention, as well as a tonic for the spleen and pancreas.

Peppermint Leaves (Mentha piperita)

Peppermint leaves stimulate bile and digestive juice secretion, improve digestion, and relieve gas pains. The

9. Yokota, 1992.

oil (menthol) helps clear mucous from the head during a cold, and calms nausea by acting as a mild anesthetic for the stomach walls. Peppermint is also good for easing tension and anxiety, as well as menstrual cramps.

Propolis

Propolis is the "glue" that honeybees use to cement their hives together. Used for thousands of years to treat wounds and ulcers, it is recommended by today's herbalists to ease sore throats and colds. Not only does it have anti-inflammatory and antiviral properties, it may also help prevent the growth of cancerous cells in the colon.[10]

Pycnogenol®

A patented blend of substances taken from the bark of the European coastal pine tree, Pycnogenol® is a powerful antioxidant. European studies have shown its effectiveness in strengthening the capillaries, increasing circulation, and preventing varicose veins. It also may help reduce the risk of skin cancer.[11]

Pygeum *(Pygeum africanum)*

A product of the African evergreen tree, pygeum has long been used to treat urinary tract problems. Controlled, double-blind studies have shown that it can reduce inflammation of the prostate and its accompanying symptoms. Although it has been studied for over twenty years and successfully used in Europe, it has only recently become available in the United States.

10. Mindell, p. 131.
11. Mayell, p. 222.

Rehmannia Root *(Rehmannia glutinosa)*

A calming and soothing tonic, Rehmannia root is a rejuvenating herb believed to cleanse the blood and act as a mild purgative. It is used by herbalists to treat blood deficiency, lack of energy, heart palpitations, insomnia, headaches, irregular menstrual periods, diabetes, and nocturnal sweats.

Rose Hips

An excellent source of bioflavonoids and vitamin C, rose hips are normally taken in supplement form or as a constituent of tea. Rose hips are potent antioxidants containing, ounce for ounce, twenty times as much vitamin C as oranges. High in vitamins B, E, K, and beta carotene, they may also have a mildly laxative or diuretic effect.

Saw Palmetto *(Serenoa repens)*

Saw palmetto berries have long been used by herbalists to treat genitourinary problems. Recent studies have shown that saw palmetto extract may help shrink enlarged prostate glands or prevent enlargement in the first place by interfering with the conversion of the male hormone testosterone to a more potent, prostate-enlarging form. This stronger form of the hormone may also be responsible for "burning" the hair roots, leading to male pattern baldness. Because it guards against the ravages of the more potent form of testosterone, some men take saw palmetto to ward off premature baldness.

Schizandra *(Schisandra chinensis)*

This Chinese herb is believed to increase stamina; relieve stress, depression, and fatigue; prolong life; and increase both sexual drive and "staying power" in men. In China, a mildly stimulating tea is made from schizandra berries. In studies on laboratory animals, schizandra helped protect the liver from toxic damage.[12] And a study of the effects of schizandra berry extract on polo horses found that aerobic capacity and overall performance were improved.[13]

Senna *(Cassia senna)*

The leaves and pods of this herb are used as an effective laxative; in fact, using senna too frequently can cause dependency. It is best when combined with an herb that has an antispasmodic effect, such as ginger. Otherwise, bowel contractions can become uncomfortably strong.

Siberian Ginseng *(Eleutherococcus senticosus)*

A completely different plant from Panax ginseng, Siberian ginseng has traditionally been used to boost energy and increase endurance. When tested on 15,350 factory workers, athletes, and others in Russia, it decreased the incidence of various diseases by 37%. The athletes, especially, enjoyed higher levels of endurance, faster running times, and quicker rates of recovery after activity.[14]

Turmeric *(Curcuma longa)*

Used as a spice in the Western world, turmeric is the source of the yellow-orange color of many curry sauces. Turmeric lowers blood cholesterol by stimulating bile production in the liver. It can also help protect against heart attacks and stroke by preventing unnecessary blood clots from forming. Its natural anti-inflammatory properties make it a natural for treating arthritis, and

12. Mindell, p. 142.
13. Mayell, p. 96.
14. Tierra, p. 231.

in Chinese medicine it is used to treat shoulder pain, menstrual cramps, and colic.

Vitamin C

Originally discovered some 250 years ago as a cure for scurvy, vitamin C is necessary for the production and maintenance of collagen, which acts as a sort of "cement" in the body, holding the cells together.

An antioxidant, vitamin C plays many important roles in the body, including assisting in wound healing and proper functioning of the immune system, protection against cancer and heart disease, and reduction of the severity of asthma attacks. It also enhances the body's absorption of iron, is important in the production of stress hormones, and may help regulate blood sugar.

Clearly, adequate intake of vitamin C is essential to maintaining good health. The recommended dietary allowance for adults for vitamin C is 60 mg per day; some green teas contain at least this much in just one cup.

White Willow Bark *(Salix alba)*

The bark of this tree has been used for centuries to relieve pain and fever—and no wonder! It contains *salicin,* a substance remarkably similar to aspirin with aspirin's ability to lessen pain and inflammation, although its effect is somewhat weaker. On the plus side, white willow bark doesn't have the unpleasant side effects of gastric irritation and bleeding often seen with aspirin. The willow also contains tannins, which aid digestion.

Now that you know what green tea (and various herbal amenities) can do for your health, let's move on to the more aesthetic aspects of tea—like savoring a hot, aromatic cup while pondering the mysteries of the universe!

CHAPTER 8

Drinking Green Tea

Tea is contentment. . . . Drinking tea, desires diminish and I come to see the ancient secret of happiness: wanting what I already have, inhabiting the life that is already mine.
—Anonymous, quoted in
TeaMind Times

Ancient Chinese poets referred to green tea as "the froth of liquid jade" or the "elixir of life." Then, in the twelfth century, the Japanese one-upped them by creating an entire art form dedicated solely to the drinking of tea—the Japanese tea ceremony (*Cha-no-yu*). Today, green tea is virtually the only kind of tea produced in Japan. It is considered so precious that less than 3% ever leaves the country. In fact, they import many times this amount to satisfy their tremendous demand.

A Question of Balance

In the Asian culture, a man who is cold or insensitive is referred to as one who has "no tea" in him, while one who is overly emotional has "too much tea" in him.

The greatest portion (80%) of Japan's tiny export crop finds its way to the United States, where it accounts for only about 4% of America's total tea intake. And the United States, in turn, imports most of its green tea from Japan—a good 4 out of every 5 pounds.[1]

Kinds of Japanese Green Tea

There are four major kinds of Japanese tea, classified according to the type of leaf it's made from, the age of the leaf, and the method used for processing. The major kinds of Japanese tea are:

• *Gyokuro* (pronounced "ghee-OH-koo-roe"), which means "gem of dewdrop" or "pearl dew." This is a precious, high-quality tea—the best. Very expensive, it is served only as a treat. (Almost no Gyokuro is exported.) To make Gyokuro, particular care is taken when cultivating the tea plants to ensure that their leaves will be especially tender and sweet. Just when the buds begin to open into leaves in April, they are carefully shaded from the strong rays of the sun by large canvases. At harvest time, only the buds of the first flush are picked—no leaves. Then, they are carefully rolled by hand (never by machines, which are too rough).

The processed Gyokuro leaves resemble fine pine needles, sharply pointed and flat. Because of their sheltered, tender treatment, the resulting brew offers a strong flavor and less bitterness than some of the lesser-quality teas, with a smooth sweet taste and a distinctly green color.

The same tenderly cared for leaves used to produce Gyokuro are air dried and left unrolled, making a product called Tencha (pronounced TEN-cha). The Tencha is then ground to a fine powder in a mortar to make Matcha, the special tea used in the Japanese tea ceremony. (Tencha is never used as is, but is always ground into Matcha.) Tencha and Gyokuro account for less than 1% of the tea produced by Japan and are rarely exported.

1. Pratt, p. 224.

• *Matcha* (pronounced "MA-cha"). This powdered version of green tea, made from ground Tencha, is dissolved in hot water and whipped to a froth with a bamboo whisk. The practice of making whipped teas from powdered leaves, which originated in China during the Sung Dynasty, was adopted by the Japanese. It is still used today in the Japanese tea ceremony; many believe that the froth created by whipping enhances the taste of the tea. *Matcha* means "liquid jade" in Japanese and this special tea is not only smooth and sweet without a trace of bitterness, but also a nourishing drink that is high in vitamin C.

• *Sencha* (pronounced "SEN-cha"). The most popular kind of tea in Japan and the one most likely to be exported to the United States, Sencha can vary greatly in price and quality. The Japanese use high-quality Sencha only on special occasions, with average quality being used on a daily basis in virtually every home or workplace. The tea leaves (bud plus top two leaves) are picked as soon as they mature, then steamed and rolled until they look like long needles. The resulting light green brew has a mixture of bitterness and sweetness and a scent that is decidedly fresh and "green."

The Mark of High Quality

Since the quality of Sencha tea varies from so-so to excellent, look for one labeled "I-Chiban Cha." This means that the tea is from the *first flush*, indicating a smoother, sweeter, less astringent brew.

• *Bancha* (pronounced "BAN-cha"). The lowest grade of Sencha, this tea is considered by the Japanese to be suitable only for children. Inexpensive and low in quality, Bancha is a pungent tea made from the large, coarse, older leaves that are pruned from the tea plant at the end of the season. Possibly because it contains less caffeine than other teas, Bancha is currently being sold as a health food product. There are two subcategories of Bancha:

• *Hojicha* (pronounced "HO-ji-cha"), made from roasted Bancha leaves, resulting in a toasted, earthy aroma and a light golden-colored brew.

• *Genmaicha* (pronounced "ghen-my-CHA"), a mixture of Bancha leaves and fire-toasted rice. This light brown brew has a savory, grainy, slightly salty taste, and is not only thirst quenching, but filling. The rice kernels sometimes pop open during shipping, giving Genmaicha its nickname: "popcorn tea."[2]

Grades of Green Tea

Green tea grades may also be listed, from highest to lowest quality, as one of the following:

• Extra Choicest
• Choicest
• Choice
• Finest
• Fine
• Good Medium
• Good Common
• Nibs
• Fannings
• Dust[3]

Kinds of Chinese Green Tea

The Chinese green teas, classified according to age and style of leaf, fall into one of three categories:

---

2. Japan Tea Exporter's Asso.; Schapira, pp. 214–218.
3. Schapira, p. 193.

• *Hoochows.* Grown in the district that bears the same name, the Hoochows are the first of China's green teas to mature in the spring. They have a light, sweet taste.

• *Pingsueys.* From the Pingsuey district in the Chekiang province, they look as appealing as the Hoochows but are not as delicious.

• *Country Greens.* This moniker is tacked on to all other green teas that are neither Hoochows nor Pingsueys. But this group boasts some of the finest of the China green teas, which are known for their clarity and richness.

There are three major ways that green tea is manufactured in China, as well as variations on those themes:

• *Gunpowder.* Called "Pearl Tea" in China, Gunpowder refers to high-quality tea leaves that are rolled into small pellets. This method of manufacturing got its name from a young English clerk who thought that the tightly rolled pellets looked like gunpowder, or perhaps more accurately, buckshot. The name is apt because each pellet "explodes" when boiling water is added and the leaves begin to unfurl. The smaller the pellets, the costlier the tea, with the highest grade deemed "extra first pinhead Gunpowder."[4]

High-quality Chinese Gunpowder tea makes a refreshing yellow-green brew with a brisk, astringent taste, while Formosan Gunpowder is sweeter with a blander taste.

• *Imperial.* This style of tea refers to older leaves that are manufactured Gunpowder style, but are less tightly rolled. (Often they have been sifted out of the regular Gunpowder tea because of their lesser quality.)

• *Young Hyson* (pronounced "HIGH-sun"). Named after the rich East India merchant who was the first to import it, this tea is made of top-quality leaves taken from wild tea trees in the Zhejiang Province. The thick,

4. McDowell, 1992.

yellow-green leaves are twisted and rolled into long, thin shapes. Young Hyson makes a stronger, more full-bodied tea than is usually found in the green tea family.

• *Hyson.* This grade of tea consists of older, poorer leaves twisted and rolled like Young Hyson. The resulting tea looks like a combination of Young Hyson and Imperial, loosely rolled and twisted.

• *Twankay.* Made from older, poorer-quality un-rolled leaves, this is the next grade lower than Hyson.

• *Hyson Skin.* Even lesser quality than Hyson or Twankay.

• *Dust.* Anything that is left over.[5]

The Best Quality Leaf

In the world's first book on tea, *Ch'a Ching*, written in the late eighth century, Lu Yu wrote that a superior tea leaf should "curl like the dewlaps of a bull, crease like the leather boots of a Tartar horseman, unfold like mist rising over a ravine, and soften as gently as fine earth swept by rain."

Brewing the Perfect Cup of Tea

No matter how high or low the quality of the tea leaves, a cup of tea can be greatly enhanced or absolutely ruined in the brewing process. But by just following a couple of simple rules, you can be assured that you'll have a delicious cup of tea every time:

1. **Choose the proper water.** The main ingredient in a cup of tea, water is the most important factor in determining its taste and aroma. Spring water is generally the preferred choice, but any good-quality bottled or filtered water will do, although you may wish to exper-

5. Pratt, p. 224.

iment with several and decide for yourself. Be aware,
however, that the wrong kind of water can ruin even
the most exquisite tea. Distilled water, water that is fluoridated or highly chlorinated, or hard water containing
large amounts of lime, magnesium, or iron can alter the
taste of the tea, so they are definitely not recommended.

2. **Boil the water.** Although the true taste of tea
cannot be fully expressed in water that is only warmed,
overboiling causes the flavor-releasing oxygen to escape,
and the resulting tea tastes flat. The best flavor results
from water that is brought just to the boiling point, and
either is poured immediately or, if the leaves are very
delicate, is just slightly cooled before pouring. This cooling can keep the leaves from "stewing" and becoming
too bitter. Generally, the higher the quality of the tea,
the longer the water should be cooled (with a maximum
of about a minute—otherwise it will be too cool). Ordi-
nary teas can take higher temperatures but should be
steeped for a shorter length of time to avoid excessive
astringency.

3. **Warm the teapot.** Before adding the tea ingredients, warm the pot with a small amount of hot water,
and then pour it out. Teacups may also be warmed this
way. (By the way, your teapot should never be subjected
to scouring powder or other harsh cleansers, which can
leave a residue that destroys the taste of the tea. Simply
rinsing the pot well after each use is sufficient.)

4. **Measure the tea.** Figure about 1.5–2 g (or 1 level
teaspoon) of loose tea per cup of water. If tea bags are
used, figure one tea bag per cup of water. Put the tea
leaves in the pot first, using either a mesh or bamboo
strainer or a wire mesh "tea ball" that can be easily
removed once steeping is completed. ("Tea balls"
should be filled only about halfway, since the leaves
expand when boiling water is added. If the tea ball is
filled up at the start, it will be too tightly packed to
infuse properly.)

5. **Steep.** Add the appropriate amount of hot (just-to-
the-point-of-boiling) water. The water causes the tea leaves

to unfold (poetically referred to as "the agony of the leaves"), releasing their essential oils and other ingredients to create the characteristic flavor, aroma and color of the tea. For best flavor, green tea leaves should be steeped for 1–3 minutes. Oversteeping can produce a bitter brew. Remember that the smaller the leaf, the more quickly the infusion is produced, and the shorter the steeping time should be. Tea bags, especially, can be filled with fannings or dust, which make very fast infusions. So unless you like drinking the juice of stewed leaves, pay strict attention to the steeping time! On the other hand, be aware that it takes at least three minutes for all the catechins in tea leaves to make their way into the liquid. It's up to you: for best flavor, steep 1–3 minutes; for greatest health benefits, steep slightly longer.

6. **Pour the tea.** Some teapots have a wire mesh screen across the neck of the teapot. This allows the loose leaves and water to mix in the pot, but prevents the leaves from pouring out through the spout. This can be very convenient, but if you have such a pot, remember that you *must* pour all of the tea out of the pot as soon as it's finished steeping, or it will continue to brew. (Not so in other pots, where you can just lift the leaves out when steeping is done.)

The Japanese believe that the tea should be poured a little at a time into each tea drinker's cup, round-robin style, until all the tea in the pot has been dispensed. That way the quality of the tea in each cup will be equal— and no one's cup will be too strong or too weak.

It's That Simple!

"Tea is nothing other than this: Heat the water, prepare the tea and drink it with propriety. That is all you need to know."

—Greatest of all Tea Masters, Senno Rikyu,
16th century

How Do You Know If It's "Good" Green Tea?

I had occasion to try a Chinese green tea that was selling for $80 a pound in Los Angeles's Chinatown. Was there any difference between this fancy tea and many of the much less expensive kinds I'd tried earlier? You bet. To begin with, the leaves were loose, maybe ½ inch long, whole (not broken), and vividly green in color and aroma. As I poured the water over the leaves, they floated to the top of the tea, then slowly opened, as if they were flowers opening during time-lapse photography. The more water the leaves took on, the heavier they became, causing them to drift gradually down to the bottom of the pot. It took about 2 minutes for all the leaves to sink—just about the time it took to complete the steeping. The tea itself was very light in color—just barely green—unlike many of the other teas I'd had that tended toward the greenish-browns. But it was the taste that was so remarkably different—much "grassier" and "greener-tasting," something akin to wet hay—with a much stronger, cleaner aftertaste. For a treat, I thought it was worth the price. But for everyday tea drinking, I knew I'd opt for something less expensive and more readily accessible.

To Add or Not to Add Milk or Honey

For reasons unknown, the Dutch began to add milk to their tea in the early 1600s. One hundred years later this practice also caught on with the French, but it was the English who truly took the habit to heart. They embellished their tea even further by adding a little sugar or honey to take the edge off the bitterness. The practice continues to this day. If you visit England and ask for your tea plain (or "black" as they call it there), your hostess (or waiter) may express surprise that anyone could possibly prefer his or her tea that way!

Milk and sugar *can* be added to green tea, if you are so inclined, but heed a word of warning: *No* self-respecting Asian would be caught dead mangling the unique flavor, aroma, and color of tea (especially green tea) with such corruptions! And from a strictly health-oriented point of view, while neither sugar nor lemon (another condiment often used with tea) affects the antioxidant action of tea, milk just might. The protein contained in milk is believed to bind up some of the antioxidants, inactivating them and making them unavailable for the body's use.[6]

Who Needs Sugar?

"Love and scandal are the best sweeteners of tea."
—Henry Fielding, *Tom Jones, 1749*

What Kind of Green Tea Offers the Most Health Benefits?

As with any crop, the quality of tea varies from year to year, field to field, and package to package. Although it is next to impossible to guarantee the amount of health-enhancing ingredients in any one cup of green tea, there *are* certain guidelines that may help ensure that you get the most for your money:

1. **Look for the higher grades of tea.** (See lists above.) Lower-quality teas are classified as such because they are made of older, coarser leaves that have remained on the bush for longer periods of time. The higher-quality teas are taken from the newest buds and the top one or two leaves, which also happen to be the leaves that have the highest polyphenol content. Higher-quality teas are also processed more quickly and carefully, which helps to preserve their polyphenols. For

6. Tuft's University Diet & Nutrition Letter.

example, the average cup of green tea contains somewhere between 40 and 90 mg of EGCg. But an analysis of a cup of Chinese Gunpowder-style tea (which is made from high-quality young leaves) shows an EGCg content of 142 mg.

Analysis of a Cup of Green Tea[7]

A cup of green tea (200 ml, Gunpowder, Hagzhou, China) contains the following:

EGCg	142 mg	
EGC	65 mg	
ECg	28 mg	
EC	17 mg	

---

2. **Use flow-through tea bags rather than flat tea bags whenever possible.** Flow-through tea bags (which look like two tea bags joined together at top and bottom) allow water to circulate through the leaves more easily, allowing them to unfold and release their catechins, essential oils, and other components more efficiently.

3. **Keep your tea in an airtight container.** The Number 1 enemy of tea freshness is moisture and the Number 2 enemy is air. Any dampness or exposure to air can degrade both the flavor and the polyphenol content of the tea. When you buy your tea loose, it might be taken from a bin and wrapped up in paper (much like fresh fish), leaving it highly vulnerable to the elements. Or it may come prewrapped in vacuum-packed foil and placed in some sort of tin. But the tins, while decorative, are rarely airtight, and once the foil is broken, the tea can become stale. Either way, for best results get an airtight, opaque plastic container and put your tea in it right away. (This also holds true for tea bags, which

7. Yang, 1993.

are often wrapped only in little paper envelopes that don't do a lot to protect the tea from the elements.) When stored properly, green tea usually has a shelf life of about six months. Stored improperly, it can lose its flavor and its health benefits much earlier.

4. **Brew the tea properly.** (*See* instructions above.) Bring fresh water to a full boil, and if you cool it, do so for only a minute. Water that isn't hot enough won't agitate the leaves sufficiently to open them up and release their active ingredients. Steep the tea leaves for the proper amount of time (one to three minutes, or see instructions on the label). And remember that most green tea leaves are good for only one infusion. Use fresh leaves every time you make a new pot.

5. **Consider buying tea that is fortified with green tea extract.** One company (Optio Health Products) has a line of green teas that contain enough green tea extract in each tea bag to provide 25 times the catechins found in other green teas. Others may provide similar benefits. Check the labels.

6. **Don't drink tea that's too hot.** Although boiling water is necessary for the proper brewing of tea, drinking tea at scalding hot temperatures increases the risk of esophageal cancer. Let it cool for a bit, then take small sips until you can drink it comfortably.

The Tea Ceremony

An ancient ritual, the tea ceremony originated in the eighth century when Lu Yu wrote his famous "everything you always wanted to know about tea" book, *Ch'a Ching*. In it he described an elaborate ceremony for the drinking of tea, complete with a strict etiquette based on Zen philosophy. This tea ceremony was so complex that it required no less than twenty-seven different pieces of equipment and two servants, making it a ritual accessible only to the rich. Not surprisingly, this particular ceremony is obsolete today.

During the Sung Dynasty (960–1280 A.D.), tea entered its "romantic age" when whipped teas became popular and were given fanciful names such as the Pure Delight, the Pearl, or Precious Thunder. Tea leaves were praised for their rarity, the cups and equipment used in the tea ceremony were works of art, and the philosophy of Zen remained king. The Japanese and Koreans established their own tea ceremonies at this time. Based on the philosophies of the Sung Dynasty, these ceremonies continue to this day. But the Chinese fell on hard times. Mongolian invaders overthrew the Sung Dynasty, established their own empire under Kublai Khan, and reigned for one hundred years. During that time, the art of tea was lost in China. When it returned much later, it was in a completely different form.

The Nine Commandments of Tea

"There are nine ways by which man must tax himself when he has to do with tea:

He must manufacture it.
He must develop a sense of selectivity and
   discrimination about it.
He must provide the proper implements.
He must prepare the right kind of fire.
He must select a suitable water.
He must roast the tea to a turn.
He must grind it well.
He must brew it to its ultimate perfection.
He must finally drink it."

—Lu Yu, *Ch'a Ching*

The Japanese Tea Ceremony

When Zen was reintroduced to Japan from China in the twelfth century, tea drinking became a widespread practice in Zen monasteries—mostly to keep the monks awake during lengthy meditation sessions! The ceremony surrounding the taking of tea was developed in the fifteenth century and became popular not only with monks but also artists, poets, and powerful rulers.

In the sixteenth century, Senno Rikyu, the greatest of all Tea Masters, accompanied the mighty warlord Hideyoshi right onto the battlefield with a small, portable teahouse that served as a place of relaxation and meditation before battle. Military leaders left their weapons outside the door of the teahouse as they gathered over a steaming bowl of tea to discuss their differences.[8] Rikyu revamped Lu Yu's elaborate, expensive tea ceremony, making it simpler and more natural so that average folk could participate as well. He applied four of the fundamental principles of Zen to the tea ceremony—harmony *(wa)*, respect *(kei)*, purity *(sei)*, and tranquillity *(jaku)*.

This ceremony, called *Cha-no-yu* (literally "the way of tea"), is an aesthetic experience that appeals to all five senses while emphasizing beauty, serenity, and relaxation of the mind. It is a disciplined ritual requiring a good deal of study and training, for every aspect of the ceremony is infused with meaning. Today the tea ceremony reaches its highest ideal only in monasteries or when performed by elite tea masters in special teahouses, although more relaxed versions are widely practiced by the middle classes.

Ideally, the ceremony takes place in a special teahouse *(sukiya)* which has been set in a garden carefully landscaped to encourage a feeling of serenity and wellbeing. The setting includes beautiful, carefully cultivated plants, a bench covered by an arbor, a stone basin for purification, plus a path made of irregular stones leading to the teahouse. Gazing at the beauty of the garden, one should be transported from the cares of everyday life to a plane of heightened awareness.

8. Republic of Tea, p. 48.

The teahouse contains two rooms—a tea room which accommodates four guests, and a service room. The door to the teahouse is approximately three feet high, causing all to bend over when entering, a sign of humility. The tea room itself is a study in tranquillity, its nine-foot-square construction based on the principles of extreme simplicity, serenity, cleanliness, and grace. The walls are earth colored, the lighting diffused. A simple flower arrangement or hanging scroll placed in the alcove of honor (the *tokonoma*) is the only decoration. Windows look out to the beautiful garden; the delicate scent of incense wafts through the air. There is no furniture—guests sit on bamboo mats on the floor.

The tea kit, which includes a teapot, water cooler, teacups, and a tray, is a very important part of the ceremony. The most favored material for this tea set (especially the teacups) is white porcelain, for it shows the natural beauty of the color of tea. Generally, the smaller the cup size, the higher the quality of the tea served.

Rules for the Japanese Tea Ceremony

Both the host and the guests at the tea ceremony are expected to conduct themselves according to the strictest rules of etiquette, many of which are some 600 years old. They include the following:

1. Those entering the tea ceremony must have clean faces, clean hands, and most importantly, clean hearts.
2. The host must greet the guests and usher them in. If he is too poor to provide them with tea or other accoutrements necessary for the ceremony, or if the food is tasteless, the guests may leave immediately.
3. The sound of boiling water (called the "soughing of the wind in the pines") prompts the ringing of the bell and the entrance of guests from the waiting room.

4. No one is allowed to speak of anything worldly at any time during the ceremony—especially politics or scandal.
5. No one, guest or host, may flatter anyone present by word or deed.[9]

Performing the Japanese Tea Ceremony

Although the tea ceremony can be carried out in many different ways (the most formal version lasts nearly four hours), most of them take place in three separate phases. In the first phase (zenseki), the windows of the tea room are covered with bamboo screens and the scroll is arranged in the alcove. When a guest enters the tea room, he or she must kneel in front of the alcove of honor and admire the scroll as well as the scent of incense in the air. The most important guest is given the seat of honor, which is both next to the host and closest to the alcove. In the second phase (nakadachi), guests are served a simple meal plus sweet cakes, after which they retire to the garden to relax. During the final, most important phase (nochiseki), the scroll is replaced by a flower arrangement, a gong is sounded, the tea utensils are brought in, and the tea is prepared and served.

The preparation and serving of the tea (temae) is a series of precise, intricate movements. Tea utensils are arranged and wiped clean, the tea bowl and whisk are warmed, and the powdered green tea (Matcha) is measured into the bowl (three heaping spoonfuls per person). Boiling water is added, then the mixture is whisked slowly and evenly until it becomes thickened. By concentrating on these movements and shutting out all worldly cares, many participants in the tea ceremony experience the same deep spiritual meaning found in meditation. Silence reigns during temae; the only sounds that can be heard are those of nature and the boiling water.

9. Schapira, p. 237.

Once the tea is made, a bowlful is passed to the principal guest, who takes a sip and compliments the host on the quality and flavor of the tea. After a few more sips, he wipes the rim of the bowl, and passes it to the next guest. Each guest repeats this ritual until all have participated. Utensils are washed and wiped and the guest of honor asks to see the tea caddy and tea scoop. The host complies with this request and leaves the room. When all guests have finished examining the tea utensils, the host comes back. Conversation regarding one of the utensils begins, and when it dies down, the fire is put out, a weak tea is served, and the ceremony concludes.

The Chinese Tea Ceremony

While the Japanese tea ceremony is lengthy, elaborate, and formal, the Chinese ceremony is shorter, more relaxed, and revolves almost entirely around the appreciation of nature. This "new" philosophy of tea drinking was developed in the fourteenth century by artists and philosophers, who were shunned by the Chinese court.

For close to one hundred years (1280–1368), China was dominated by Mongol invaders. During that time, the arts of calligraphy, painting, sculpture, and tea simply faded from the scene. But once the Ming Dynasty drove out the Mongols in 1368, an attempt was made to reestablish these lost arts. Unfortunately, the new court was made up of outlaws and other unsavory types who had little interest in such things. Artists, scholars, and philosophers found themselves retreating to the mountains for inspiration. There they mingled with hermits and began to incorporate the philosophies of these nature lovers into works of art. Thus began the "naturalist" period of tea, which is the basis of the modern Chinese tea ceremony.

Every aspect of the Chinese tea ceremony symbolizes

these mountain retreats. The teahouse is a thatched or wooden hut, like those of the hermits. Incense represents the scents of nature. A painting of an outdoor scene or a poem about nature written on a scroll symbolizes the inspiration found in the great outdoors. Music represents the sound of the wind or the singing of the birds, and a flower arrangement symbolizes nature's flora and fauna.

In keeping with this "natural" theme, earthenware pots and cups in muted tones are used for preparing and serving the tea. Whole tea leaves are used rather than whipped powder. Everything is reminiscent of the earth and nature—nothing must remind the guests of the modern day. (Man-made materials such as plastic are strictly taboo.)

Rules for the Chinese Tea Ceremony[10]

The Chinese tea ceremony is much less rule-bound than the Japanese, but there are certain points of etiquette that must be observed. Among them:

1. Guests should engage in general discussions about art, poetry, philosophy, or tea, without arguing or debating.
2. No one should dominate the conversation.
3. The host must make sure that no guest sits without tea in his or her cup for more than a short period of time.
4. When pouring water, the host must not spill even a drop.
5. For the first cup, guests use two hands; for all other cups, they use one.
6. The right hand is always used—never the left, except when two hands are used during the first cup. The reason for this: In ancient days, the right

10. Courtesy of Erik LaPort, Ten Ren Tea Culture Foundation.

hand carried the weapon. By occupying this hand with a teacup, one showed that he had no intent of harming anyone. The left hand, however, which was used to clean oneself, was better left on the lap!

The Way to Enlightenment

"Tea with us became more than an idealization of the form of drinking: It was a religion of the art of life. The beverage grew to be an excuse for the worship of purity and refinement, a sacred function. . . . The tea room was an oasis in the dreary waste of existence where weary travelers could meet to drink from the common spring of art appreciation. The ceremony was an improvised drama whose plot was woven about the tea, the flowers, and the paintings. Not a color to disturb the tone of the room, not a sound to mar the rhythm of things, not a gesture to obtrude on the harmony, not a word to break the unity of the surroundings, all movements to be performed simply and naturally—such were the aims of the tea ceremony. And strangely enough it was often successful."

—Okakuro Kakuzo,
The Book of Tea, 1906

Serenity in a Stressed-Out World

The Japanese have believed for centuries that health and longevity are promoted by the drinking of tea. And while scientists all over the world have confirmed that the tea leaf really *does* contain health-promoting substances, let's not forget that even the processes of making and drinking tea surely have beneficial effects. The health benefits of boiling water, adding tea leaves, inhaling the fragrant aroma, sitting down to sip the tea, relaxing, and taking a break from the stresses of life should not be underestimated.

Stress is the plague of modern man, an invisible killer that contributes to heart disease, stroke, cancer, diabetes, impaired immune system response, and a host of other dangerous conditions. It also prompts the release of highly charged chemicals in the body such as *epinephrine, norepinephrine,* and *catecholamine,* which raise blood sugar, release fats into the bloodstream, and break down muscle tissue. Over time, stress can exhaust the body's resources, leaving one more and more vulnerable to disease and debilitation. Clearly, stress is a major factor in many illnesses and deaths. Finding a way to handle stress is, therefore, one key to better health.

When scientists studied more than 3,000 Tokyo women over the age of fifty who regularly practiced the tea ceremony, they found that these women lived longer than those in a matched control group who did not engage in the ceremony.[11] Was it the ingestion of tea catechins that was responsible, or was it the release of stress? No one knows for sure. What we do know is that relaxing and taking a break from life has been a part of the tea experience from the start. And undoubtedly, we can all benefit by stopping to take a regular "breather." Perhaps the serenity that we all seek is closer than we think, and can be found in a cup of steaming hot green tea during a few stolen moments in a favorite chair.

Ah, the Simple Things in Life!

"Surely everyone is aware of the divine pleasures which attend a wintry fireside: candles at four o'clock, warm hearthrugs, tea, a fair tea-maker, shutters closed, curtains flowing in ample draperies to the floor, whilst the wind and rain are raging audibly without."
—Thomas De Quincey,
Confessions of an English Opium-Eater, 1822

---

11. Sadakata, 1992.

CHAPTER 9

Where Can I Buy Green Tea?

Tea is drunk to forget the din of the world.
—T'IEN YIHENG

As news of its incredible health benefits begins to spread, green tea should become easier and easier to find. Right now it can be purchased in health food stores and Asian markets, and some brands can even be found in grocery stores. (For an explanation of the health benefits of many of the ingredients added to the teas, *see* Chapter 7.)

Here is a list of green teas that are currently sold in markets or health food stores. Any added ingredients are also listed, as well as a taste description. If you're interested in purchasing any of these teas and can't find them locally, you may wish to contact the manufacturers directly.

Teas Purchased in Retail Outlets

Alvita Products, Inc.
600 East Quality Drive
American Fork, UT 84003
800-258-4828

- *Chinese Green Tea.* Called an "antioxidant rich blend," this tea, according to the manufacturer, provides 100% of the RDA for vitamin C, while its orange and lemon peel extracts provide bioflavonoids and citrus terpenes. Probably owing to all of those vitamin C–rich additions, the brew is rather tart, but a little sweetening may be all it needs. This blend also comes in lemon, lime, orange, and tangerine flavors.

Alvita has also come up with a new line of tea blends called RemeTeas™ aimed at treating special health conditions. Although no claims are made about their effectiveness, you can tell by their names (and their ingredients) what they're supposed to do. No fewer than eleven different RemeTeas™ contain green tea:

- *Caribbean Breathabilitea™.* Contains green tea, peppermint, ma huang, lobelia, turmeric, and licorice.
- *Ivory Coast Sip-N-C+™.* Contains green tea, bilberry, vitamin C, citrus bioflavonoids, Pycnogenol®, and grape skin.
- *Mediterranean Detoxitea™.* Contains green tea, artichoke, milk thistle, turmeric, schizandra, vitamin C, angelica, kudzu, and astragalus.
- *Gulf Stream Prosti-Brew™.* Contains green tea, saw palmetto, Korean ginseng, pygeum, soy extract, and pumpkin seed.
- *Scandinavian Winter Comfort™.* Contains green tea, echinacea, goldenseal, elderberry, astragalus, propolis, licorice, ginger, white willow bark, and vitamin C.
- *Indian Arth-Right™.* Contains green tea, turmeric,

boswellia serrata, ginger, white willow bark, fever-few, Devils' claw, and licorice.

- *Lancaster County Migra-Wonder*™. Contains green tea, feverfew, white willow bark, and ginger.
- *Pacific Coast Slimmer*™. Contains green tea, chromium picolinate, ginger, cayenne, and Citrimax™.
- *Chinese Mellow Magic*™. Contains green tea, kava kava, schizandra, and chamomile.
- *Himalayan Sennalax*™. Contains green tea, senna, cascara sagrada, aloe vera, and peppermint.
- *Manchurian Brain Blend*™. Contains green tea, gingko biloba, Korean ginseng, and ma huang.

AriZona Beverages
1212 Sycamore Street
Cincinnati, OH 45210
800-TEA-3775

- *Green Tea with Ginseng and Honey.* The only bottled green tea I've come across, this tea is worth the price for the packaging alone! A statuesque light green bottle adorned with pink cherry blossoms, this green tea contains honey, high fructose corn syrup, and ginseng extract. It's sweet and quite pleasant, but green tea aficionados will find it hard to believe this sweet beverage is the same one they're used to drinking.

R.C. Bigelow, Inc.
201 Black Rock Turnpike
Fairfield, CT 06430
203-334-1212

- *Japanese Green Tea.* This delicious tea makes a clear, light green brew that more closely resembles the tea served in Japanese restaurants than many of the teas sampled.

Celestial Seasonings, Inc.
4600 Sleepytime Drive
Boulder, CO 80301-3292
800-525-0347

- *Emerald Gardens Green Tea.* A fragrant combination of green tea, Ceylon tea (a black tea), orange blossoms, and ginger root, plus the flavors of plum and passionfruit. The Ceylon tea is added to "smooth out" the natural astringency of this green tea, and the addition of plum and passionfruit make it a fruity and aromatic brew.
- *Herbal Comfort Antioxidant Assurance Green Tea.* One cup of this brew provides 100% of your daily vitamin C requirement and contains hibiscus, Siberian ginseng root, roasted chicory root, alfalfa, licorice root, vitamin C, carrots, ginger root, beta carotene, and vitamin E. Its lemony-orange flavor is a bit tart, but leaves your mouth with a very fresh feeling.

Good Earth Teas
831 Almar Avenue
Santa Cruz, CA 95060
408-459-8818

- *Green Tea Blend.* This green tea is a blend of tea leaves, lemongrass, and natural flavors, resulting in an aromatic, fruity brew with a slightly bitter aftertaste.

Maitake Products, Inc.
P.O. Box 1354
Paramus, NJ 07653
800-747-7418

- *Green Tea (Matcha) and Maitake Mushroom.* This is a blend of the powdered Japanese tea used in the tea ceremony and Maitake, the medicinal mushroom that contains the polysaccharide β 1.6 Glucan, an immune system booster. The brew is surprisingly tasty, producing a musky, earthy flavor and a light brown color.

Optio Health Products, Inc.
500 Citadel Drive, #120
Los Angeles, CA 90040
800-678-4692

All of the Optio teas contain Polyphenon 60, a high-powered green tea extract (50:1 at a standardized 60% polyphenols[1]). According to the manufacturer, each cup of tea is twenty times more potent than the average green tea.

- *Supreme Green Tea.* Gold in color, this tea tastes clean and green, and contains green tea leaves, green tea extract, and lemon powder. It doesn't taste particularly lemony though—it simply tastes like good green tea.
- *Ginkgo Plus Green Tea.* This delicious mint-flavored brew never seems to get bitter, no matter how long you steep it. In addition to the green tea leaves and extract, it contains ginkgo biloba extract (50:1) and peppermint leaves.
- *Antioxidant Plus Green Tea.* This tea contains rose hips, beta carotene, blueberry leaves, bilberry extract, green tea leaves, and green tea extract. The result is a light brown brew with a slightly metallic taste.
- *Weight Loss Plus Green Tea.* Although it doesn't taste a lot like green tea, this orange-and-cinnamon-flavored drink is quite delicious and refreshing. It contains green tea leaves and extract, cinnamon, orange peel, gymnema sylvestre extract and ginger. Studies show that gymnema sylvestre helps block the sensation of sweet taste, while reducing the absorption of sugar into the bloodstream—just the thing for weight watchers.

---

1. *See* the Appendix for a discussion of extracts.

- *Ginseng Plus Green Tea.* Ah yes, the unmistakable rooty taste of panax ginseng! Luckily, this brew makes it palatable with the addition of peppermint and licorice root. As a result, it's really not bitter at all and the licorice leaves a nice fresh feeling in your mouth.

Republic of Tea
8 Digital Drive, Suite 100
Novato, CA 94949
800-298-4TEA

- *Big Green Hojicha.* This roasted green tea comes the closest to tasting like coffee of any tea I've tasted yet, but without a trace of bitterness. Nutty, almost smoky, it is surprisingly delicious and satisfying.
- *Moroccan Mint.* There's something about mint and green tea that makes them natural partners. The mint adds a refreshing aroma and a hint of sweetness without masking the flavor of the tea.

Seelect Herb Tea Co.
P.O. Box 1969
Camarillo, CA 93011
800-273-3532

- *Green Tea.* A clean, clear, light green brew with mild astringency and a refreshing taste.

The Stash Tea Co.
P.O. Box 910
Portland, Oregon 97207
800-547-1514

- *Premium Green Tea.* A plain yet satisfying green tea with good body and a light greenish brown color.

Traditional Medicinals
c/o Natural Resources
6680 Harvard Drive
Sebastopol, CA 95472-5121
800-747-0390

- *Golden Green Tea.* This green tea contains lemongrass, giving it a slightly lemony flavor and a very fresh aftertaste.

Triple Leaf Tea, Inc.
P.O. Box 421572
San Francisco, CA 94142
800-552-7448

- *Green Tea.* Refreshing and bracing, this tea is the real thing—just tea leaves, nothing added. The resultant brew is a greenish-golden color with a satisfying, delicious, and mildly astringent taste.
- *Jasmine Green Tea.* This light and fragrant green tea really smells like flowers, and its yellow-green brew goes down smoothly without a hint of bitterness.

Uncle Lee's Tea
11020 Rush Street
South El Monte, CA 91733
818-350-3309

- *Green Tea.* This plain green tea is pleasantly full-bodied and bracingly astringent.
- *Jasmine Green Tea.* The addition of jasmine flowers to green tea gives a floral aroma and sweetness that lightens the tea's natural tartness.
- *Green Tea—Tropical Fruit Flavor.* Its aroma may remind you of tutti-frutti gum, but it's pleasant and goes down smoothly.
- *Green Tea—Cinnamon Apple Flavor.* Spicy and slightly sweet tasting, this is a good tea for a cold day.
- *System Builder.* This blend of green tea, vitamin C,

and herbs has a slight orangy flavor that goes well with the tea's natural astringence.

- *Energy Booster*. This green tea is combined with ginseng (which is believed to increase energy and vitality) and other herbs that just may be able to get you going in the morning. The taste is brightened by the addition of ginger and lemon.
- *Tox Guard*. A cranberry-flavored blend of green tea, milk thistle seed, and other herbs, the tartness of this tea is actually rather refreshing. The addition of a little sugar makes it taste something like diluted fruit juice.

The Yogi Tea Company
2545 Prairie Road
Eugene, OR 97402
800-225-3623

- *Green Tea with Kombucha and Chinese Herbs*. This tea has a definite fruity quality paired with a refreshing hint of licorice. It has a strong aroma and a fine taste (although far from the taste of traditional green tea). Besides green tea leaves, it contains Kombucha (the "fungus" purported to cure a host of ills), lemongrass, spearmint leaf, ginseng, licorice root, Pai Shu root, ginger root, Eucommia bark, Royal Jelly, cinnamon bark, Ling Chih mushroom, Dong Quai root, Rehmannia root, and lycii fruit.
- *Green Tea with Cat's Claw and Kombucha*. This tea contains everything found in the Chinese herb blend plus an extract of cat's claw bark, which is believed to boost the immune system. The taste and aroma are similar (or identical) to the Chinese herb tea.
- *Green Tea with Panax Ginsengs and Kombucha*. Strong, rooty, and bitter, even the addition of spearmint, licorice, ginger, and cinnamon can't mask the distinctive taste of ginseng root. Contains

all the ingredients of the Chinese herb blend plus nine different ginseng root extracts and astragalus root.

- *Green Tea with Triple Echinacea and Kombucha (with Elderberry)*. This tea has the ingredients listed above plus a triple echinacea extract *(Echinacea pallida, Echinacea augustifolia,* and *Echinacea purpurea* root), elderberry, and goldenseal root. Unfortunately, the addition of all of these roots give the tea a bitterness not unlike the Panax ginsengs blend.

Mail-Order Sources

If you're having trouble locating green tea or you're looking for the pricier brands, check out the Chinatown section of your nearest big city or contact one of the mail-order manufacturers listed below.

Eastrise Trading Corporation
318 South Date Avenue
Alhambra, CA 91803
888-288-TEAS

Eastrise offers a wealth of green teas including Japanese (Sencha, Genmaicha, and the difficult-to-find Gyokuro) and Chinese (Country Green, Young Hyson, and several kinds of Gunpowder) as well as various special Jasmines. They also offer no less than thirty-two different rare green teas, ranging in price from $5.50 to $58.00 per pound. Write or call for a complete list of teas and prices.

Frontier Bulk Teas
3021 78th Street
Norway, IA 52318
800-669-3275

Frontier offers several green teas that are worth looking into, including Dragonwell (also known as Lung-ching, a fine Chinese green tea), Sencha, Young Hyson, Gunpowder, and Gunpowder Pearl Mint (flavored with spearmint and peppermint leaves). They also offer a sweet-smelling Jasmine tea, which is made by spreading jasmine flowers over dried green tea leaves. As the flowers dry, they impart a delicious scent to the tea leaves. Another version of this tea, Jasmine Spice, is made by adding orange peel, cinnamon, cloves, and cardamom.

Gold Mine Natural Food Co.
3419 Hancock Street
San Diego, CA 92110-4307
619-296-8536

This mail-order house caters to those interested in macrobiotic and/or organic foods. As such, it offers a host of Ohsawa® teas distributed by the company that was started by George Ohsawa, one of the pioneers of macrobiotics. These teas are grown without chemicals or fertilizers, and include toasted Bancha, Sencha, and Genmaicha (using 100% organic brown rice). And although not a tea in the strictest sense of the word (only the leaves of the *Camellia sinensis* bush make true tea), "teas" made from lightly roasted one-year-old twigs, or a combination of twigs and leaves, are also offered. These twig "teas" have an interesting, smoky flavor that is quite pleasant and unusual. The Goldmine catalog (which contains a lot more than tea) is available upon request.

Silk Road Teas
P.O. Box 287
Lagunitas, CA 94938
415-488-9017

Silk Road Teas specializes in Chinese teas, offering a selection of more than 200 different green teas. Those who aren't sure what kinds to try can opt for a sampler of six green teas at the very reasonable price of about

$20. (Each of the six 15-gram packets makes twelve 8-ounce pots of tea.) Call or write for a catalog.

SpecialTeas, Inc.
500 Summer Street, Suite 404
Stamford, CT 06901
888-365-6983

This company specializes in fine green teas from China and Japan ranging in price from $7.10 to $29.00 per half pound. The China Greens include a delicious tea called Pi Lo Chun, which is grown among peach, plum, and apricot trees and seems to have absorbed their fragrances. (It was formerly called "Astounding Fragrance.") Their Japan Greens include Bancha, Sencha Fine and Extra Fine, Genmaicha, and Gyokuro Extra Fine. Purchases can be made by mail, by phone, or through the Internet at http://www.specialteas.com/.

Ten Ren Tea and Ginseng Co., Inc.
75 Mott Street
New York, NY 10013
800-292-2049

This tea company offers both Japanese and Chinese green teas, either loose or bagged, with prices ranging from $4.00 for a box of tea bags to $125.00 for a pound of top-grade tea. Besides the branch listed above, Ten Ren has stores in California, Illinois, and Queens, New York.

Where to Buy Matcha

The powdered tea that is whipped to a froth for use in the Japanese tea ceremony is typically quite hard to find. Mail-order houses usually don't carry it because the demand is low, it's expensive, and many people don't care for the flavor. (It's an acquired taste.) If you're lucky, you might be able to find it in certain

Asian markets. (In Los Angeles, I had to make the trek downtown to Little Tokyo, the Japanese version of Chinatown, before I could find it. Even then, it was only in one market and they had only one kind.)

Information on Tea Culture

To find out more about Chinese tea ceremonies; tea philosophy, art, and history; or tea classifications and quality judging, contact:

Ten Ren Tea Culture Foundation
Professor J. Erik LaPort
111 West Garvey Avenue
Monterey Park, CA 91754
818-288-2012
818-288-4121 (fax)

CHAPTER 10

Green Tea Recipes

Tea is a work of art and needs a master hand to bring out its noblest qualities.

—OKAKURA KAKUZO,
The Book of Tea, 1906

Although green tea is at its most delicious and satisfying when served hot and unadorned, it can be a delightful addition to other recipes. Its delicate flavor is not over-powering, so it can blend well with fruit juices to make a refreshing drink or add its own subtle but luscious taste to ice cream. Try some of these suggestions for delicious, health-boosting additions to your diet:

Iced Drinks

Green Tea Mintade

During the sweltering dog-days of summer, your body needs plenty of liquids to keep its cooling system in peak form. And what could be more refreshing than a combination of green tea, ice, and mint?

| 2 bunches or handfuls of | ¼ cup honey |
| fresh mint | ¼ cup lemon juice |

**4 cups prepared green
    tea**

Wash mint and place in saucepan. Add 1 cup green
tea and the honey. Bring to a boil and simmer uncovered
for 10 minutes. Chill, then strain mint syrup. Add lemon
juice and remaining green tea to mint syrup. Pour over
ice in tall glasses and, if desired, garnish with mint sprigs
and lemon slices. Makes 4 tall or 6 punch cup servings.

Green Tea Lemonade

*An old standby with a fresh new twist. Sugar-frosted glasses
make it even more special.*

**1 can (12 ounces) frozen
    lemonade
    concentrate, thawed**

**4 ½ cups prepared green
    tea**

Combine lemonade concentrate and green tea, mixing well. Refrigerate. Serve in sugar-frosted glasses. (Dip
rim of glass in lemon juice, then in sugar. Put in freezer
for at least 10 minutes before filling with tea.) Garnish
with a sprig of mint. Makes 12 half-cup servings.

Tropical Green Tea Julep

*This recipe combines Asia, Polynesia, and the Deep South
in an exotic and glamorous drink sure to elicit enthusiastic
comments from guests.*

**2 cups diced ripe papaya
2 cups diced pineapple
2 cups prepared green
    tea
¼ cup lemon juice
¼ to ⅓ cup honey**

**Cracked ice
Papaya cubes, kiwi slices,
    and maraschino
    cherries
4–6 wooden skewers**

Combine papaya, pineapple, green tea, lemon juice, and honey in blender. Puree at high speed until liquefied. Pour over cracked ice in tall glasses. Garnish with "kabobs" made of papaya cubes, kiwi slices, and maraschino cherries speared on wooden skewers. Makes 4 to 6 servings.

Green Tea Float

Steaming hot green tea poured over vanilla ice cream makes a melted, creamy dessert drink that's something like liquefied green tea ice cream. Truly worthy of the title "divine elixir of the gods"!

1 cup prepared green tea, steaming hot	2 scoops vanilla ice cream Sprigs of mint

Place ice cream in a tall glass; pour hot tea over it. Add mint sprig to garnish. Makes 1 serving.

Fruity Iced Green Tea

A simple, pretty way of dressing up iced green tea without changing its original flavor.

4 cups prepared green tea, chilled Ice cubes made from fruit juice (such as apple, grape, cranberry, or orange)	Fruit kebabs—your choice of fruit chunks (such as grapes, strawberries, pineapple, or kiwi) on wooden skewers

Place fruit juice ice cubes into tall glasses; pour tea over them. Garnish with fruit kebabs. Makes 4 servings.

Punches

Green Tea Party Punch

Green tea's natural astringency blends perfectly with citrus juices, giving this easy punch a refreshing lilt.

2 cups honey, preferably orange blossom or clover
3 cups water
1 cup mint leaves, packed
1 cup orange juice
1 cup lemon juice
8 cups prepared green tea
Block of ice
Slices of lemon and orange

Combine honey and water in a saucepan and stir over medium heat until dissolved. Bring to a boil, add mint, and simmer 5 minutes. Cool and stir. Combine with orange and lemon juices and green tea. Chill thoroughly. Pour punch over ice in a punch bowl and garnish with lemon and orange slices. Makes 24 half-cup servings.

Apricot Tea Punch

This delicious peach-colored punch combines the clean freshness of green tea with apricot nectar and ginger ale. The result is a light, bubbly drink appropriate for any gathering, from casual to elegant.

1 quart prepared green tea
3 cups apricot nectar
2 cups orange juice
½ cup lemon juice
½ cup granulated sugar
1 bottle (1 liter) ginger ale, chilled
Ice cubes

In a pitcher or other container, combine hot tea, apricot nectar, orange juice, lemon juice, and sugar. Mix well. Refrigerate until chilled.

At serving time, combine chilled tea mixture with ginger ale in a large punch bowl. Add ice as needed to keep the punch cool. Makes 30 half-cup servings.

Fruity Green Tea Punch

This crimson punch is perfect for the holidays, yet refreshing enough to serve in the middle of summer.

9 cups water	2 cups orange juice
9 fresh mint leaves	2 cups lemon juice
3 cups granulated sugar	2 cups cherry juice blend
4 cups prepared green	or apple-cherry juice
tea	2 cups pineapple juice

In a large saucepan, combine water and mint leaves and simmer for 5 minutes. Remove mint leaves and add sugar to the mint-flavored water. Boil for 5 minutes, then let syrup cool.

In a large container, combine sugar syrup, green tea, orange juice, lemon juice, cherry juice blend, and pineapple juice. Mix well. Let mixture stand at room temperature for 1 hour, then refrigerate until ready to serve. Makes 44 half-cup servings.

Black Cherry Tea Punch

This luscious punch combines black cherries, green tea, cinnamon, and ginger, creating a sweet and spicy drink guaranteed to make your guests feel special.

2 cups pitted fresh or frozen sweet black cherries	1 stick (2 inches) cinnamon, broken into small pieces
6 cups green tea, prepared and refrigerated	¼ cup fresh lemon juice
	1 cup granulated sugar, or to taste
1 teaspoon chopped fresh ginger	

In a saucepan, combine cherries and 2 cups of pre-pared green tea. Bring to a boil, then reduce heat, cover, and simmer for 15 minutes. Set mixture aside to cool.

In another saucepan, combine remaining 4 cups of prepared tea, ginger, and cinnamon; bring to a boil. Let cool. Strain to remove ginger and cinnamon.

Place cooked cherries in a sieve and drain off juices, bruising fruit gently in order to get as much flavor as possible into the juice. Drain 20 minutes or longer. Discard bruised cherries.

Combine cherry juice with strained mixture; add lemon juice and sugar. Mix well. Refrigerate until ready to serve. Makes about 18 half-cup servings.

Hot Drinks

Apricot-Orange Tea

Tea is at its most comforting when hot, and the addition of some apricot nectar, lemon peel, and brown sugar can be just the thing on a cold night.

3 cups water	6 green tea bags
1 cup apricot nectar	3 tablespoons firmly
4 strips lemon peel (each	packed brown sugar
1 inch long)	

In a medium saucepan, bring water, apricot nectar, and lemon peel to a boil. Simmer covered for 2 minutes. Remove from heat and add tea bags. Cover and steep for 5 minutes. Remove tea bags and lemon peel; stir in sugar. Pour into teacups and garnish, if desired, with additional lemon peel. Makes 4 7-ounce servings.

Hot Apple Tea

Hot spiced cider is an old favorite, especially around Christmas. Try adding the subtle shading of astringency to the brew by popping in a few green tea bags.

1 quart apple juice	6 vanilla beans
4 green tea bags	6 twists of orange or
6 cinnamon sticks *or*	lemon rind

Bring apple juice to a boil. Pour over tea bags in a teapot, cover, and brew 2 or 3 minutes. Serve with cinnamon stick or vanilla bean and orange or lemon rind in each cup or mug. Makes 6 5-ounce servings.

Spiced Green Tea

In Sweden, "glogg" is made for St. Lucia's Day celebrations by combining fruit juices, spices, and plenty of aquavit, a super high-potency liquor. Here we skip the booze and substitute green tea, creating a hot drink that's even tastier, and a lot better for your health.

6 green tea bags	1 tablespoon whole
6 cups boiling water	allspice
1 ½ cups orange juice	1 tablespoon whole
1 ½ cups pineapple juice	cloves
¼ cup granulated sugar	2 sticks cinnamon
¼ cup firmly packed	2 vanilla beans
brown sugar	Orange slices, for
2 tablespoons honey	garnish

In a large container, steep tea bags in boiling water for 5 minutes. Remove and discard tea bags. Add orange juice, pineapple juice, granulated sugar, brown sugar, honey, allspice, cloves, cinnamon sticks, and vanilla beans. Mix well.

Pour into a slow cooker; heat on warm setting 2 to 3 hours. Serve hot, garnished with orange slices. Makes about 10 1-cup servings.

Pineapple-Green Tea

I like to take a big icy-cold thermos of this delightful drink to the beach on a hot summer's day.

1 ½ cups water
½ cup pineapple juice
2 green tea bags

2 tablespoons firmly
packed dark brown
sugar

In a small saucepan, bring water and pineapple juice to a boil. Remove from heat and add tea bags. Cover and steep for 3–4 minutes. Remove tea bags; stir in sugar. Makes 2 8-ounce servings.

Moroccan Green Tea

During Moroccan feasts, guests sit on embroidered pillows, sampling endless rounds of exotic foods as they watch belly dancers shimmy and shake. But the culmination of the evening is a cup of delicious, refreshing, mint-flavored green tea.

3 green tea bags
1 handful fresh mint
  leaves or ¼ teaspoon
  mint extract

3 cups boiling water

Place tea bags and mint leaves or extract in teapot; add boiling water. Steep for 3 minutes. If fresh mint leaves are used, strain. Makes 3 servings.

Desserts

Green Tea Ice Cream

Anyone who frequents Japanese restaurants will be familiar with this luscious, slightly musky-tasting ice cream. Now you can make it yourself.

**1 pint vanilla ice cream   1–1 ½ teaspoon Matcha
                                (powdered green tea)**

Soften ice cream slightly. Add Matcha and beat mixture until well blended. Freeze until firm. Makes 4 ½-cup servings.

Green Tea—Mango Sorbet

The sweet, tropical taste of mangos combines with the herbaceousness of green tea and the surprising explosion of ginger. A true adventure for the taste buds and the perfect climax for a Japanese or Chinese meal.

**¾ cup sugar   ½ cup fresh lime juice
1 cup prepared green tea   3 tablespoons ginger,
6 mangos, peeled and   peeled and minced
  diced**

Place sugar and prepared green tea in a small saucepan. Bring to a boil. Reduce heat, simmer 5 minutes. Set aside to cool to room temperature.

Puree mango with lime juice and ginger. Combine with cooled sugar water mixture.

Pour into a metal 13 x 9-inch pan. Freeze 1 hour. Using a sturdy fork, break up ice to slushy consistency. Repeat this step 3 times at 1-hour intervals. Each time the sorbet will be firmer. After the final freeze, use an electric mixer, food processor, or whisk to get a good final texture. Pack into a storage container, cover, and freeze. Makes 12 ½-cup servings.

"So hear it then, my Rennie dear,
  Nor hear it with a frown;
You cannot make the tea so fast
  As I can gulp it down.
I therefore pray thee, Rennie dear,
  That thou wilt give to me
With cream and sugar softened well,
  Another dish of tea!"
—Dr. Samuel Johnson,
  extemporized for his friend Boswell

❧

Appendix

Choosing a Green Tea Extract

What's an Extract?

To make an extract, the key ingredient(s) of a plant are isolated and drawn out, using water or steam, then condensed before spray drying. All the leaves, stems, cellulose, water, and extra components are discarded, leaving a much more compact version of the sought-after ingredients in powder form. In the case of green tea, it's the health-promoting catechins that are extracted. The resulting powder can be put into tablet or capsule form or made into a liquid. In laboratory tests using green tea and animals, extracts are used almost exclusively because they are easy to measure and administer. (It's hard to get a rat to drink ten cups of tea!)

Extract Strength

Choosing an extract can be tricky because it's difficult to know just what you're getting. Most extracts will show a ratio on their labels indicating potency. This ratio shows how much raw herb was used to produce the extract. For example, a 50:1 green tea extract means that 50 pounds of dried leaves were used to produce 1 pound of dry extract, while a 5:1 extract indicates that only 5 pounds of dried leaves were used to make the same amount of extract. As you can see, the higher the first number in the ratio, the stronger the product. When buying green tea extract, a 50:1 ratio is optimal. Although a higher ratio would be more potent, the price at this point begins to get extremely steep.

Standardization

Since the health benefits of green tea are primarily due to the action of the catechins, many green tea extracts will list the catechin content as a percentage on their labels. For example, a *60% catechin content* means that 60% of the dry weight of the extract is made up of catechins. In other words, for every pound of extract, there are 9.6 ounces (60% of 16 ounces) of pure catechins. Some extracts may also list the amount of EGCg that they contain, since EGCg is the most potent of the catechins. This is also expressed as a percentage of the total dry weight of the extract. So if the extract contains 60% catechins and 30% EGCg (which falls into the catechin category), you can read it as: 60% catechins, half of which is EGCg.

To make sure that you're truly getting the amounts listed on the label, look for the word "standardized." Green tea leaves, like any crop, can be young or old, fresh or stale, from rich or poor soil and therefore can contain varying amounts of catechins. That's why *standardization* was invented—a way to guarantee that the amount of a particular compound would always be at a certain level. To produce a standardized extract, scientific testing is conducted at several points during the extraction process. The goal is to eliminate any variability and ensure that the concentration of ingredients remains consistent. With a standardized extract, you *always* get the listed percentage, no matter what. But without the word *standardized* on the label, you might be getting less.

How Much to Take?

In the average cup of green tea, there may be anywhere from 50 to 100 mg of catechins. Many of the studies done on green tea have concluded that a daily intake of 3–10 cups of green tea (the equivalent of 300–1,000 mg of catechins, using the higher amount) is necessary to achieve certain health benefits. According to Dr. Yukihiko Hara, director of Food Research Labs at Mitsui Norin Co. Ltd. in Japan and the distinguished author of several scientific studies on green tea, to get the minimum amount of catechins (300 mg) from an extract, you'd need about 480 mg of a 50:1 extract that contains 60% catechins. (60% of 480 mg = 300 mg). If you're taking an extract with the same percentage of catechins but a lower ratio, then you'd need to increase the dose to get the same amount of catechins. Unfortunately, many liquid extracts don't tell you what their catechin percentage is, or they don't list their strength.

In a more perfect world, manufacturers would give us a break from the guessing game by listing catechin amounts on their product labels. Although the liquid extracts are notorious for their lack of information, many green tea extracts in capsule or tablet form do list their *polyphenol* content. (For example, Natures Herbs contains 50 mg polyphenols per capsule, Kal Inc. 36 mg of polyphenols, Solgar's Green Tea Vegicap 60 mg of polyphenols, and Solgar's Antioxidant Formula 10 mg of polyphenols.) It's important to remember, however, that *polyphenol* content and *catechin* content are two different things. Catechins are a *subgroup* of polyphenols, so whatever the polyphenol content of a supplement may be, you can be sure that the catechin content is less. You might consider taking half again as many milligrams of polyphenols as the desired amount of catechins (i.e., 450 mg of polyphenols to get 300 mg of catechins). Obviously this is a very rough estimate, but it may be the best you can do considering the sketchy information available.

As you can see, figuring out how to get the desired amount of green tea catechins from an extract is quite difficult and confusing. Unfortunately, until manufacturers begin to offer green tea extracts with the catechin contents clearly printed on their labels, this confusion will continue to reign. Writing or calling extract manufacturers to request that they change their current labeling practices may help to start the ball rolling in the right direction.

Glossary

ACE (Angiotensin converting enzyme) The release of this enzyme causes the tiny muscles surrounding the arteries to clamp down, making the arteries smaller and driving up blood pressure. Preventing this "clamping down" of the muscles and keeping the arteries from narrowing is an important step in preventing high blood pressure.

Activation The second stage of cancer development, in which an initiated cell suddenly begins to multiply uncontrollably, forming a mass of new tissue called a tumor.

Aflatoxin A substance produced by a mold that grows on peanuts that is one of the world's most potent carcinogens.

Amylase An enzyme produced by the pancreas that is responsible for breaking apart the large, complex starch molecule into glucose molecules that can be used by the body as fuel. Blocking the action of amylase results in the inability of the body to use the starch molecule as a source of energy.

Antioxidants Substances—such as catechins, vitamin C, beta carotene, vitamin E, and selenium—that block free radical damage to the cells. Antioxidants can help prevent cancer, heart disease, and other degenerative diseases while slowing the aging process by blocking certain destructive reactions in the body.

Bancha The lowest grade of Sencha, Bancha is a pungent tea made from the large, coarse, older leaves that are pruned from the tea plant at the end of the season.

Black tea Leaves of the *Camellia sinensis* bush that are withered, broken, fermented, and dried.

Caffeine A compound found in coffee, tea, and kola nuts used medicinally as a stimulant and diuretic.

Camellia sinensis An evergreen shrub or tree, the leaves of which are used to make tea.

Cancer A malignant tumor that grows uncontrollably, invading other tissues and bodily systems.

Carcinogen Any substance that produces or incites cancer.

Catechins A member of the polyphenol group and its subgroup, the flavonoids, catechins are found in abundance in green tea. These compounds are powerful disease fighters and potent antioxidants with a host of beneficial effects, from preventing food spoilage to halting the progression of cancer. The catechins found in green tea include *gallocatechin (GC)*, *epicatechin (EC)*, *epigallocatechin (EGC)*, *epicatechin gallate (ECg)*, and *epigallocatechin gallate (EGCg)*.

Cholesterol A waxy, fatty substance that is manufactured in the liver and found in all animal tissues. Cholesterol is used in many different ways in the body: to build cell membranes, as an insulating sheath around nerve fibers, and as a basis for certain hormones. It is also one of the major ingredients in plaque, and too much cholesterol in the blood can cause great amounts of plaque to be deposited on artery walls.

Coronary artery disease (CAD) The blocking of the arteries that feed the heart muscle (usually due to excess plaque in the blood) which can lead to the death of heart tissue (a heart attack).

Country Green A group of Chinese green teas that includes some of China's finest; known for their clarity and richness.

Diabetes A condition in which glucose in the blood cannot enter the cells to be utilized for energy. No matter how "hungry" the cells may be, the glucose continues to float by in the bloodstream. A buildup of blood glucose causes major damage to the body over time and can result in kidney failure, blindness, gangrene, stroke, and heart disease.

DNA Various nucleic acids in the cell that dictate the cell's structure and function. Substances that bind to the DNA can radically change the way a cell behaves.

EGCg Epigallocatechin gallate, the catechin with the most potent antioxidant capacity. EGCg is responsible for most of green tea's health benefits.

Fermentation An enzymatically controlled breakdown of a substance. In the case of tea, polyphenols are broken down by the enzyme polyphenol oxidase.

Flavonoids A group of over 200 plant pigments that have powerful antioxidant properties and are helpful in treating allergic inflammation, fragile capillaries, and bleeding gums. A subgroup of the polyphenols, flavonoids are found in green tea, leafy green vegetables, and the outer layers and peels of fruits and vegetables.

Fluoride A mineral found in tea that interacts with tooth enamel, hardening it and making it 50–70% less susceptible to decay.

Flush   The development of new leaves and buds on the tea plant. The first flush usually occurs in spring.

Free radicals   Unstable molecules that travel around the body looking for electrons to "steal" from other molecules, wreaking havoc on cells, tissues, and systems. Free radicals are thought to be a major cause of cancer, heart disease, and aging.

Genmaicha   Tea made from a mixture of bancha leaves and fire-toasted rice. Sometimes called "popcorn tea."

Glucan (dental plaque)   A sticky, water-insoluble substance that accumulates on the teeth and is produced by the combination of *Streptococcus mutans* bacteria and sugars in the mouth.

Green tea   Leaves of the *Camellia sinensis* bush that are steamed or pan-fired immediately after plucking to halt the enzymatic breakdown of the polyphenols. Leaves are then rolled, twisted, and dried.

Gunpowder   High-quality green tea leaves from China that are rolled into small pellets.

Gyokuro   The highest quality of Japanese green tea, Gyokuro is made up of only the buds of the first flush, which are carefully rolled by hand.

HDL (High-density lipoproteins)   The "good" cholesterol, the form that carries cholesterol away from the arteries and out of the body.

Hojicha   Tea made from roasted Bancha leaves, resulting in a toasted, earthy aroma and a light golden-colored brew.

Hoochow   The first of China's green teas to mature in the spring, these have a light, sweet taste and a pleasing appearance.

Hypertension   Also known as high blood pressure, this "silent killer" is one of the biggest warning signs of heart disease, indicating that the heart is working too hard to pump the blood through the circulatory system. High blood pressure can also lead to cracks or tears in the blood vessels, prime spots for clot formation. Hypertension is a major cause of coronary artery disease, congestive heart failure, heart attacks, and strokes.

Hyson This grade of Chinese green tea consists of older, poorer leaves that are twisted and rolled like Young Hyson.

Imperial This style of Chinese green tea contains older leaves that are manufactured Gunpowder style, but are less tightly rolled.

Initiation The first part of the cancer process, in which carcinogenic substances break into a healthy cell and "hijack" its DNA, altering the "instruction manuals" that tell the cell how to behave.

Insulin A hormone produced by the pancreas that makes it possible for blood glucose to enter a cell to be used as energy.

Insulin receptor site An area on the cell where insulin "docks," like a key fitting into a lock. If the site becomes blocked (usually by fat cells), insulin can't attach and glucose can't enter the cell. This blocking is a common cause of diabetes.

Kidney stone An accumulation of calcified material that lodges in a duct in the kidney.

LDL (Low-density lipoprotein) The "bad" cholesterol, the form that carries cholesterol to artery walls and deposits it there.

Lu Yu An eighth-century poet and scholar who wrote *Ch'a Ching (Classic of Tea)*, and became the patron saint of tea. In his three-volume work, he described everything that was then known about tea: the origins of the tea plant, the varieties of tea, the methods of tea cultivation and production, the benefits of tea drinking, and even precise instructions for brewing and serving tea.

Matcha Powdered green tea that is used today primarily in the Japanese tea ceremony.

Nitrosamine A powerful inducer of stomach cancer.

Oolong tea Leaves of the *Camellia sinensis* bush that are partially fermented, making the finished product a cross between green and black tea.

Peroxidation The process in which oils are turned rancid owing to exposure to oxygen. Peroxidation of the fats in the brain is thought to be a major cause of brain aging.

Pingsuey Green teas that originate in the Pingsuey district of China's Chekiang province. They look as appealing as the Hoochows but are not as pleasant tasting.

Plaque A fatty substance made up of cholesterol, fat, blood clots, and/or cellular debris that can accumulate on artery walls. If the accumulation becomes too thick, blood supply can be cut off, resulting in a heart attack or stroke.

Platelets Small cells in the blood that clump together to form a clot in response to injury. Too much clumping, however, can cause unwanted clots that may bring on a heart attack or stroke.

Polyphenol A group of naturally occurring plant compounds that are powerful antioxidants and may help fight cancer, heart disease, and other disease states in the body.

Polyphenol oxidase An enzyme present in fresh tea leaves that combines with oxygen when the leaf is plucked and begins to change the structure of the tea polyphenols from catechins to thearubigens and theaflavins.

Sencha The most popular kind of tea in Japan and the one most likely to be exported to the United States,

Sencha can vary greatly in price and quality. The Japanese use high-quality Sencha only on special occasions, with average quality being used on a daily basis in virtually every home or workplace.

Senno Rikyu   The greatest of all Tea Masters, Rikyu devised seven rules for the Japanese tea ceremony in the sixteenth century that are still in effect today. He made the formerly elaborate and expensive tea ceremony accessible to the middle class.

Singlet oxygen   One of the most common and most destructive of the free radicals.

Stroke   The death of a portion of the brain tissue due to the blockage of a blood vessel.

Tea ceremony   A centuries-old ritual for drinking tea originating in China that revolves around simplicity, cleanliness, serenity, grace, and the appreciation of nature.

Tencha   The same tenderly cared for leaves used to produce Gyokuro are air dried and left unrolled to make this product. Tencha is never used as is; it is always ground to a powder to make Matcha.

Theaflavins and thearubigens   Compounds made from the oxidation of catechins when tea leaves are fermented to make black tea. They also have antioxidant properties, although in most cases not as strong as those of the green tea catechins.

Thromboxane   A substance released by the blood's platelets that causes them to clump together to form a clot. Thromboxane also causes the constriction of the blood vessels.

Total cholesterol   The measure of the sum of all kinds of cholesterol (HDL, LDL, and others) in an individual's blood at a given moment, expressed in milligrams per deciliter of blood.

Tumor A mass formed by cells that have multiplied uncontrollably. Some tumors are cancerous, while others are not and may not be an immediate threat to the health.

Young Hyson Top-quality leaves taken from wild tea trees in the Zhejiang Province of China that are twisted and rolled into long, thin shapes.

Bibliography

Adachi K, Nariba H, Juroda H: Potential of host-mediated antitumor activity in mice by beta-glucan obtained from *Grifola frondosa* (maitake). Chem Pharm Bull 35:262–270, 1987.

Ali M, et al. Prostaglan Leukotr Fatty Acids 40:281, 1990.

Block G: Epidemiologic evidence regarding vitamin C and cancer. Am J Clin Nutr 54:1310S–14S, 1991.

Blot, WJ, Li JY, Taylor PR: Nutrition intervention trials in Linxian, China: supplementation with specific vitamin/mineral combinations, cancer incidence and disease specific mortality in the general population. J Natl Cancer Inst. 85:1483–1492, 1993.

Carlin BI, Pretlow TG, Pretlow TP, Mukhtar H, Mohan RR, Agrawal R, Resnick MI: Green tea polyphenols inhibit growth of prostate cancer xenograft CWR-22 and decrease ornithine decarboxylase activity: implications for prostate cancer chemoprevention. Taken from the Internet, 11/27/96.

Chen J: The effects of Chinese tea on the occurrence of esophageal tumors induced by N-nitrosomethylbenzylamine in rats. Prev Med 21:385–391, 1992.

Chisaka T, Matsuda H, Kubomura Y, Mochizuki M, Yamahara J, Fujimura H: The effect of crude drugs on experimental hypercholesterolemia: Mode of action of (-)-epigallocatechin gallate in tea leaves. Chem Pharm Bull 36(1):227–233, 1988.

Conney A, Wang Z, Huang M, Ho C, Yang C: Inhibitory effect of green tea on tumorigenesis by chemicals and ultraviolet light. Prev Med 21:361–369, 1992.

Curhan GC, Willett WC, Rimm EB, Spiegelman D, Stampfer MJ: Prospective study of beverage use and the risk of kidney stones. Am J Epidemiol, 143:3, 1996.

Food Research Laboratories, Mitsui Norin Co., Ltd. Prophylactic functions of green tea polyphenols, Chemco Industries, Inc., 1993.

Food Research Laboratories, Mitsui Norin Co., Ltd. Tea and health, n.d.

Forster K: Tea types and their processing in China. Tea Coffee Trade J 162:26–32, 1990.

Fox A, Fox B: *Alternative Healing*. Franklin Lakes, NJ: Career Press, 1996.

Fox B: *Foods to Heal By*. New York: St. Martin's Paperbacks, 1996.

Fujiki H, Yoshizawa S, Horiuchi T, Suganuma M, Yatsunami J, Nishiwaki S, Okabe S, Nishiwaki-Matsushima R, Okuda T, Sugimura T: Anticarcinogenic effects of (-)-epigallocatechin gallate. Prev Med 21:503–509, 1992.

Gebner B, Voelp A, Klasser M: Study of the long-term action of a ginkgobiloba extract on vigilance and mental performance as determined by means of quantitative pharmaco-EEG and psychometric measurements. Arzneim-Forsch 35:459–465, 1985.

Goo YU, McLaughlin JK, Blot WJ, Ji BT, Dai Q, Fraumeni JF: Reduced risk of esophageal cancer associated with green tea consumption. J Natl Cancer Inst 86(11):855–858, June 1, 1994.

Goto R, et al. Jpn J Cancer Clin Spec 344:1990.

Graham HN: Green tea composition, consumption, and polyphenol chemistry. Prev Med 21:334–350, 1992.

Green MS, Harari G: Association of serum lipoproteins and health-related habits with coffee and tea consumption in free-living subjects examined in the Israeli CORDIS study. Prev Med 21:532–545, 1992.

Hainer RM: Studies of copper chlorophyline–odorant systems. Science 119:609–610, 1954.

Hamilton EM, Whitney EN, Sizer FS: *Nutrition: Concepts and Controversies, 3d ed.* St. Paul: West Publishing Co., 1985.

Hara, Y: Effect of tea polyphenols on the intestinal flora. Up to Date Food Processing: 28(2), Feb. 1993.

Hara Y: The effects of tea polyphenols on cardiovascular diseases. Paper presented to the First International Symposium on the Physiological and Pharmacological Effects of *Camellia sinensis* (tea), New York, March 4–5, 1991.

Hara, Y, Honda M: The inhibition of α-amylase by tea polyphenols. Agric Biol Chem 54:1939–1945, 1990.

Harler CR: *The Culture and Marketing of Tea.* London: Oxford University Press, 1964.

Hatta H, Skanaka S, Tsuda N, Kanatake H, Yamamoto T, Ebina T: Antirotavirus agent in green tea. Thirty-seventh Annual Meeting of Japanese Society of Virologists (Abstract, p. 327), Osaka, Japan, 1989.

Hattori M, Kusumoto IT, Namba T, Ishigami T, Hara Y: Effect of tea polyphenols on glucan synthesis by glucosyltransferase from *Streptococcus mutans*. Chem Pharm Bull 38(3):717–720, 1990.

Hertog MGL et al.: Dietary antioxidant flavonoids and risk of coronary heart disease: The Zutphen Elderly Study. Lancet 342:1007–1011, 1993.

Hikino H, Kiso Y, Hatano T, Yoshida T, Okuda T: Anti-hepatotoxic actions of tannins. J Ethnopharmacol 14:19, 1985.

Hindmarch I, Subhan Z: The psychopharmacological effects of ginkgobiloba extract in normal healthy volunteers: Int J Clin Pharmacol Res 4:89–93, 1984.

Ho C, Chen Q, Huang BS, Zhang K, Rosen R: Antioxidative effect of polyphenol extract prepared from various Chinese teas. Prev Med 21:520–525, 1992.

Horiba N, Maekawa Y, Ito M, Matusumoto T, Nakamura H: A pilot study of Japanese green tea as a medicament: Antibacterial and bactericidal effects. J Endodontics 17(3):122–124, 1991.

Hu Z, Toda M, Okubo S, Hara Y, Shimamura T: Mitogenic activity of (-)-epigallocatechin gallate on B-cells and investigation of its structure-function relationship. Int J Immunopharmac 14(8):1399–1407, 1992.

Imai K, Nakachi K: Cross sectional study of effects of drinking green tea on cardiovascular and liver diseases. Brit Med J 310:693–696, Mar 18, 1995.

Ishigami T, Hara Y: Anti-carious and bowel modulating actions of tea. Food Research Laboratories, Mitsui Norin Co., Ltd. Shizuoka, Japan, n.d.

Ito Y, Ohnishi S, Fujie K: Chromosome aberrations induced by *aflatoxin B1* in rat bone marrow cells in vivo and their suppression by green tea. Mutation Res 222:253–261, 1989.

Jain AK, Shimoi K, Nakamura Y, Kada T, Hara Y, Tomita I: Crude tea extracts decrease the mutagenic activity of N-methyl-N'-nitrosoguanidine in vitro and in intragastric tract of rats. Mutation Res 210:1–8, 1989.

John TJ, Mukundan P: Virus inhibition by tea, caffeine and tannic acid. Ind J Med Res 69:542–545, 1979.

Joy T: Green tea manufacture: Japanese style. Tea Coffee Trade J 158:22–23, 1986.

Kada T, Kaneko K, Matsuzaki S, Matsusaki T, Hara Y: Detection and chemical identification of natural bio-antimutagens. A case of the green tea factor. Mutation Res 150:127–132, 1985.

Kahn S, Katiyar S, Agarwal R, Mukhtar H: Enhancement of antioxidant and phase II enzymes by oral feeding of green tea polyphenols in drinking water to SKH-1 hairless mice: Possible role in cancer chemoprevention. Cancer Res 52: 4050–4052, July 15, 1992.

Kanaya S, Goto K, Hara Yoshio, Hara Yukihiko: The physiological effects of tea catechins on human volunteers. Study done at Seirei Mikatabara General Hospital, Fujieda, Shizuoka Pref. 426, Japan.

Kato I, Tominaga S, Matsuura A, Yoshii Y, Shirai M, Kobayashi S. A comparative case-control study of colorectal cancer and adenoma. Jpn J Cancer Res 81:1101–1108, 1990.

Keli SO, Hertog MGL, Feskens EJM, Kromhout D: Dietary flavonoids, antioxidant vitamins, and incidence of stroke. Arch Intern Med 156:637–642, Mar. 25, 1996.

Klaunig JE: Chemopreventive effects of green tea components on hepatic carcinogenesis. Prev Med 21:510–519, 1992.

Kono S, Ikeda M, Tokudome S, Kuratsune M: A case-control study of gastric cancer and diet in northern Kyushu, Japan. Jpn J Cancer Res (Gann) 79:1067–1074, 1988.

Kono K: The decolonization of Methicillin-resistant *Staphylococcus aureus* in the respiratory tract by inhalation of tea catechin. School of Medicine, Fukuoka University, Japan, 1992.

Kono S, Shinchi K, Ikeda N, Yanai F, Imanishi K: Green tea consumption and serum lipid profiles: a cross-sectional study in northern Kyushu, Japan. Prev Med 21:526–531, 1992.

Liu L, Castonguay A: Inhibition of the metabolism and genotoxicity of 4-(methylnitrosamino)-1-(3-pyridyl)-1-butanone (NNK) in rat hepatocytes by (+)-catechin. Carcinogenesis 12:1203–1208, 1991.

Lou F, Zhang M, Zhang X, Liu J, Yuan W: A study on tea pigment in the prevention of atherosclerosis. Paper presented to the First International Symposium on the Physiological and Pharmacological Effects of *Camellia sinensis* (tea), New York, March 4–5, 1991.

Matsuzaki T, Hara Y: Antioxidative activity of tea leaf catechins. Nippon Nogeikagaku Kaishi (59)129–134, 1985.

Mayell M: *Off-the-Shelf Natural Health*. New York: Bantam Books, 1995.

McDowell I, Owuor P: The taste of tea. New Scientist 11:30–33, Jan. 1992.

Mindell E: *Earl Mindell's Anti-Aging Bible*. New York: Fireside Books, 1996.

Mori A, Hiramatsu M, Yokoi I, Edamatus R: Biochemical pathogenesis of post-traumatic epilepsy. Pavlovian J Bio Sci 25(2):54–62, Apr. Jn. 1990.

Mukhtar H, Wang Z, Katiyar S, Agarwal R: Tea components: antimutagenic and anticarcinogenic effects. Prev Med 21:351–360, 1992.

Mukoyama A, Ushijima H, Nishimura S, Koike H, Toda M, Hara Y, Shimamura T: Inhibition of rotavirus and enterovirus infections by tea extracts. Jpn J Med Sci Biol 44:181–186, 1991.

Muramatsu K, Fukuyo M, Hara Y: Effect of green tea catechins on plasma cholesterol level in cholesterol-fed rats. J Nutr Sci Vitaminol 32:613–622, 1986.

Murray MT: *Encyclopedia of Natural Medicine.* Rocklin, CA: Prima Publishing, 1991.

Murray MT: *The Healing Power of Foods.* Rocklin, CA: Prima Publishing, 1993.

Nakamura Y, Harada S, Kawase I, Matsuda M, Tomita I: Inhibition of in vitro neoplastic transformation by tea ingredients. Paper presented to the First International Symposium on the Physiological and Pharmacological Effects of *Camellia sinensis* (tea), New York, March 4–5, 1991.

Nakane H, Ono K: Differential inhibitory effects of some catechin derivatives on the activities of human immunodeficiency virus reverse transcriptase and cellular deoxyribonucleic and ribonucleic acid polymerases. Biochemistry 29:11, 1990.

Nakayama M, Toda M, Okubo S, Shimamura T: Inhibition of influenza virus infection by tea. Lett Appl Microbiol 11:38–40, 1990.

Nariba H: Working paper: Anti-diabetic activity by maitake mushroom *(Grifola frondosa),* 1994.

Oguni I: *Green Tea and Human Health.* Japan Tea Exporters' Association, Shizuoka, Japan, n.d.

Oguni I, Nasu K, Kanaya S, Ota Y, Yamamoto S, Nomura T: Epidemiological and experimental studies on the antitumor activity by green tea extracts. Jpn J Nutr 47:93–102, 1989.

Oguni I, Cheng SJ, Lin PZ Hara U: Protection against cancer risk by Japanese green tea. Prev Med 21:332, 1992.

Ohtsuru M: Anti-obesity activity exhibited by orally administered powder of maitake mushroom *(Grifola frondosa)*: Anshin 198, July 1992.

Perdue L: *The French Paradox.* Renaissance Publishing, Sonoma, CA, 1992.

Prasad KN: Modulation of the effects of tumor therapeutic agents by vitamin C. Life Sci 27(4):275–80, 1980.

Pratt JN: *Tea Lover's Treasury.* The Cole Group, Santa Rosa, CA, 1982.

Republic of Tea: *The Book of Tea & Herbs.* The Cole Group, Santa Rosa, CA, 1993.

Sadakata S, Fukao A, Hisamichi S: Mortality among female practitioners of Chanoyu (Japanese "tea-ceremony"). Tohoku J Exp Med 166:475–477, 1992.

Sagesaka-Mitane Y, Miwa M, Okada S: Platelet aggregation inhibitors in hot water extract of green tea. Chem Pharm Bull 38(3):790–798, 1990.

Sakagami H, Asano K, Hara Y, Shimamura T: Stimulation of human monocyte and polymorponuclear cell iodination and interleukin-1 production by epigallocatechin gallate. J Leuk Biol, 1992.

Sakamoto K, et al.: Green tea linked to positive DNA effect on rats. Paper presented to the Federation of American Societies for Experimental Biology (FASEB) meeting, Anaheim, CA, April 24–28, 1994.

Sakanaka S, Kim M, Taniguchi M, Yamamoto T: Antibacterial substances in Japanese green tea extract against

Streptococcus mutans, a cariogenic bacterium. Agric Biol Chem 53(9):2307–2311, 1989.

Sato Y, Nakatsuka H, Watanabe T, Hisamichi S, Shimizu H, Fujisaku S, Ichinowatari I, Ida Y, Suda S, Kato K, Ikeda M: Possible contribution of green tea drinking habits to the prevention of stroke. Tohoku J. Exp. Med. 157:337–343, 1989.

Schapira J, Schapira D, Schapira K: *The Book of Coffee & Tea,* 2d rev. ed. New York: St. Martin's Griffin, 1996.

Shibata A, Mack TM, Paganini-Hill An, Ross RK, Henderson BE: A prospective study of pancreatic cancer in the elderly. Int J Cancer 58:46–49, 1994.

Shiraki M, et al: Antioxidative and antimutagenic effects of theaflavins from black tea. Mutation Res 323:29–34, 1994.

Sohn OS, Surace A, Fiala ES, Richie JP, Colosimo S, Zang E, Weisburger JH: Effects of green and black tea on hepatic xenobiotic metabolizing systems in the male F344 rat. Xenobiotica 24(2):119–127, 1994.

Stensvold I, Tverdal A, Solvoll K, Foss OP: Tea consumption. Relationship to cholesterol, blood pressure and coronary and total mortalilty. Prev Med 21:546–533, 1992.

Tajima K, Tominaga S: Dietary habits and gastro-intestinal cancers: a comparative case-control study of stomach and large intestinal cancers in Nagoya, Japan. Jpn J Cancer Res (Gann) 76:705–716, 1985.

Tea Council of the U.S.A., Health benefits of black tea. New York, n.d.

Terada A, Hara H, Nakajyo S, Ichikawa H, Hara Y, Fukai K, Kobayashi Y, Mitsuoka T: Effect of supplements of tea polyphenols on the caecal flora and caecal metabolites of chicks. Microbial Ecol in Health and Disease 6:3–9, 1993.

Theodosakis J, Adderly B, Fox B: *The Arthritis Cure.* New York: St. Martin's Press, 1997.

Tierra M: *The Way of Herbs.* New York, NY: Pocket Books, 1990.

Toda M, Okubo S, Hiyoshi R, Shimamura T: The bactericidal activity of tea and coffee. Lett Appl Microbiol 8:123–125, 1989.

Toda M, Okubo S, Ikigai H, Suzuki T, Suzuki Y, Hara Y, Shimamura T: The protective activity of tea catechins against experimental infection by *Vibrio cholerae* O1. Microbiol Immunol 36(9):999–1001, 1992.

Uchida S, Edamatus R, Hiramatus M, Mori A, Nonaka G, Nishioka I, Niwa M, Oaki M: Condensed tannins scavenge oxygen free radicals. Med Sci Res 15:831–832, 1987.

Uchida S, Ohta H, Niwa M, et. al.: Prolongation of lifespan of stroke-prone hypertensive rats. Chem Pharm Bull 38 (4):1049–1052, 1990.

Ukers WH: *All About Tea.* Tea & Coffee Trade Journal, New York, 1935.

Wang Z, Cheng SJ, Zhou ZC, Athar M, Khan WA, Bickers DR, Mukhtar H: Antimutagenic activity of green tea polyphenols. Mutation Res 223:273–285, 1989.

Wang Z, Huang M, Ferraro T, Wong C, Lou Y, Reuhl K, Iatropoulos M, Yang C, Conney A: Inhibitory effect of green tea in the drinking water on tumorigenesis by ultraviolet light and 12-*O*-tetradecanoylphorbol-13-acetate in the skin of SKH-1 mice. Cancer Res 52:1162–1170, March 1, 1992.

Wang Z, Huang M, Ho C, Chang R, Ma W, Ferraro T, Reuhl K, Yang C, Conney A: Inhibitory effect of green tea on the growth of established skin papillomas in mice. Cancer Res 52:6657–6665, December 1, 1992.

Wang Z, Huang MT, Lou YR, Xie JG, et al.: Inhibitory

effects of black tea, green tea, decaffeinated black tea and decaffeinated green tea on ultraviolet B light-induced skin carcinogenesis in 7, 12 dimethylbenz(a)-anthracene-initiated SKH-1 mice. Cancer Res 54:3428–3435, 1994.

Wang Z, Khan W, Bickers D, Mukhtar H: Protection against polycyclic aromatic hydrocarbon-induced skin tumor initiation in mice by green tea polyphenols. Carcinogenesis 10:4110–415, 1989.

Weatherstone J: Historical introduction. In *Tea: Cultivation to consumption*. Eds. Willson KC, Clifford MN. London: Chapman & Hall, 1992, 1–23.

Wei J, et al.: Mental stress-induced myocardial ischemia and cardiac events. J Amer Med Assoc 275:1651–1656, 1996.

Weisburger JH: On the role of tea in modifying causes of major human cancers. Paper presented to the First International Symposium on the Physiological and Pharmacological Effects of *Camellia sinensis* (tea), New York, March 4–5, 1991.

Wellness Encyclopedia: Eds. the Editors of the University of California, Berkeley Wellness Letter. Boston: Houghton Mifflin Co., 1991.

Xu Y, Ho C, Dhimant D, Chung F: Effects of green tea and its components on lung tumorigenesis induced by a tobacco-specific nitrosamine. Paper presented to the First International Symposium on the Physiological and Pharmacological Effects of *Camellia sinensis* (tea), New York, March 4–5, 1991.

Yang CS, Wang Z: Tea and cancer. J Natl Cancer Inst 85(13):1038–1049, 1993.

Yokota M, Koseikai Clinic, Tokyo, Japan: Observatory trial at anti-obesity activity of maitake mushroom *(Grifola frondosa)*. Anshin, 202, July 1992.

Yokoyama T: A cup of humanity sharing with you, now. Japan Tea Exporters' Association, Shizuoka, Japan, n.d.

Yoshino K, et al. Antioxidative effects of black tea theaflavins and thearubigens on lipid peroxidation of rat liver homogenates induced by *tert*-butyl hydroperoxide. Bio Pharmacol Bull, 17(1): 146–149, 1994.

Yu G, Hsieh C, Wang L, Shun-zhang Y, Xue-liang L, Tie-hua J: Green-tea consumption and risk of stomach cancer: a population-based case-control study in Shanghai, China. Cancer Causes and Control 6:532–538, 1995.

Zhao B, Li X, He R, Cheng S, Wenjuan X: Scavenging effect of extracts of green tea and natural antioxidants on active oxygen radicals. Cell Biophys 14:175–185, 1989.

Zheng W, Doyle TJ, Kushi LH, Sellers TA, Hong C, Folsom AR: Tea consumption and cancer incidence in a prospective cohort study of postmenopausal women. Am J Epidemiology 144(2): 175–182, 1996.

ABOUT THE AUTHOR

Nadine Taylor, M.S., R.D., a registered dietitian, is the coauthor of several articles on health and nutrition. She has conducted seminars throughout the country on women's health issues, eating disorders, and other nutritionally related subjects. She has a special interest in alternative healing and natural remedies. Her book *If You Think You Have an Eating Disorder* . . . will be published in early 1998.

EAT HEALTHY WITH KENSINGTON

COOKING WITHOUT RECIPES
by Cheryl Sindell   (1-57566-142-X, $13.00/$18.00)
Unleash your creativity and prepare meals your friends and family will love with the help of this innovative kitchen companion. COOKING WITHOUT RECIPES includes intriguing culinary strategies and nutritional secrets that will stir your imagination and put the fun back into cooking.

EAT HEALTHY FOR $50 A WEEK
Feed Your Family Nutritious, Delicious Meals for Less
by Rhonda Barfield   (1-57566-018-0, $12.00/$15.00)
Filled with dozens of recipes, helpful hints, and sample shopping lists, EAT HEALTHY FOR $50 A WEEK is an indispensable handbook for balancing your budget and stretching your groceries while feeding your family healthy and nutritious meals.

THE ARTHRITIC'S COOKBOOK
by Collin H. Dong, M.D.   (1-57566-158-6, $9.95/$12.95)
and Jane Banks
Afflicted with debilitating, "incurable" arthritis, Dr. Collin H. Dong decided to fight back. Combining traditional Chinese folk wisdom with his western medical practice, he created a diet that made his painful symptoms disappear. Today, used in conjunction with regular arthritis medications, this groundbreaking diet has provided thousands of Dr. Dong's patients with active, happy, and virtually pain-free lives. It can do the same for you.